Health and Medicine in the Indian Princely States

Since the 1980s there has been a continual engagement with the history and the place of Western medicine in colonial settings and non-Western societies. In relation to South Asia, research on the role of medicine has focused primarily on regions under direct British administration. This book looks at the 'Princely states' that made up about two-fifths of the Subcontinent. Two comparatively large states, Mysore and Travancore – usually considered as 'progressive' and 'enlightened' – and some of the Princely states of Orissa – often described as 'backward' and 'despotic' – have been selected for analysis. The authors map developments in public health and psychiatry, the emergence of specialized medical institutions, the influence of Western medicine on indigenous medical communities and their patients, and the interaction between them.

Exploring contentious issues currently debated in the existing scholarship on medicine in British India and other colonies, this book covers the 'indigenization' of health services, the inter-relationship of colonial and indigenous paradigms of medical practice, and the impact of specific political and administrative events on and changes in health policies. The book also analyzes British medical policies and the Indian reactions and initiatives they evoked in different Indian states. It offers new insights into the interplay of local adaptations with global exchanges between different national schools of thought in the formation of what is often vaguely, and all too simply, referred to as 'Western' or 'colonial' medicine.

A pioneering study of health and medicine in the Princely states of India, it provides a balanced appraisal of the role of medicine during the colonial era. It will be of interest to students and academics studying South Asian and imperial and commonwealth history; the history of medicine; the sociology of health and healing; and medical anthropology, social policy, public health, and international politics.

Waltraud Ernst is Professor in the History of Medicine at Oxford Brookes University, UK.

Biswamoy Pati is a historian and teaches at the Department of History, Delhi University, and is presently a Senior Fellow at the Nehru Memorial Museum and Library, New Delhi, India.

T.V. Sekher is Professor in the Department of Population Policies and Programs at the International Institute for Population Sciences (IIPS), Deemed University, Mumbai, India.

Routledge Studies in South Asian History

11 **Bureaucracy, Community and Influence in India**
Society and the State, 1930s–1960s
William Gould

12 **A History of State and Religion in India**
Ian Copland, Ian Mabbett, Asim Roy, Kate Brittlebank and Adam Bowles

13 **Hindu Mahasabha in Colonial North India, 1915–1930**
Constructing Nation and History
Prabhu Bapu

14 **Cinema, Transnationalism, and Colonial India**
Entertaining the Raj
Babli Sinha

15 **Environment and Pollution in Colonial India**
Sewerage Technologies along the Sacred Ganges
Janine Wilhelm

16 **The Kashmir Conflict**
From Empire to the Cold War, 1945–66
Rakesh Ankit

17 **Hindu Nationalism, History and Identity in India**
Narrating a Hindu Past under the BJP
Lars Tore Flåten

18 **The Formation of the Colonial State in India**
Scribes, Paper and Taxes, 1760–1860
Hayden J. Bellenoit

19 **Health and Medicine in the Indian Princely States**
1850–1950
Waltraud Ernst, Biswamoy Pati and T.V. Sekher

Health and Medicine in the Indian Princely States

1850–1950

Waltraud Ernst, Biswamoy Pati
and T.V. Sekher

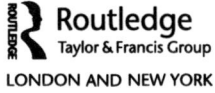 Routledge
Taylor & Francis Group

LONDON AND NEW YORK

First published 2018
by Routledge
2 Park Square, Milton Park, Abingdon, Oxon OX14 4RN

and by Routledge
711 Third Avenue, New York, NY 10017

Routledge is an imprint of the Taylor & Francis Group, an informa business

British Library Cataloguing-in-Publication Data
A catalogue record for this book is available from the British Library

Library of Congress Cataloging-in-Publication Data
Names: Ernst, Waltraud, 1955– author. | Pati, Biswamoy, author. |
    Sekher, T. V., author.
Title: Health and medicine in the Indian princely states : 1850–1950 / Waltraud
    Ernst, Biswamoy Pati and T.V. Sekher.
Other titles: Routledge studies in South Asian history ; 19.
Description: Abingdon, Oxon ; New York, NY : Routledge, 2018. | Series:
    Routledge studies in South Asian history ; 19 | Includes bibliographical
    references and index.
Identifiers: LCCN 2017002092 | ISBN 9780415679350 (hardback) |
    ISBN 9781315165875 (ebook)
Subjects: MESH: Public Health Administration—history | Delivery of Health
    Care—history | Mental Health Services—history | Health Policy—history |
    Colonialism—history | History, 19th Century | History, 20th Century | India
Classification: LCC RA418.3.I4 | NLM WA 11 JI4 | DDC 362.10954—dc23
LC record available at https://lccn.loc.gov/2017002092

ISBN: 978-0-415-67935-0 (hbk)
ISBN: 978-1-315-16587-5 (ebk)

Typeset in Times New Roman
by Apex CoVantage, LLC

Contents

List of figures   viii
List of tables   ix
About the authors   x
Acknowledgements   xi

Introduction   1
WALTRAUD ERNST, BISWAMOY PATI, AND T.V. SEKHER

SECTION 1
Mysore   11
T.V. SEKHER

1   **Plague administration in Princely Mysore:**
    resistance, riots, and reconciliation   13

    Administrative measures to control plague   14
    Public resistance   19
    Plague and riots: the Ganjam case   21
    Discussion and conclusion   22

2   **Addressing public health and sanitation in Mysore,**
    1881–1921: 'model' state and 'native' administrators   26

    Organization of public health administration   27
    Organization of Sanitary Department   31
    Epidemic administration: vaccination   33
    Administering an epidemic: the case of influenza
       pandemic of 1918   36
    Concluding observations   37

SECTION 2

The Orissan states 43

BISWAMOY PATI

3 **Princely maladies: leprosy** 45

'The empire strikes back' 46
Colonial 'unreason' and ways of explaining leprosy 48
Leprosy: the Adivasi healing system and the
Princely state of Keonjhar 50
Mayurbhanj 55
Conclusion 56

4 **Smallpox in the Princely enclaves of Orissa** 61

Smallpox and the world of the tribals 62
Smallpox and the colonial establishment 65
The Princely states 69
    Gangpur 70
    Mayurbhanj 70
    Keonjhar 71
    Kalahandi 72
    Nilgiri 73
    Dhenkanal 73
Conclusion 74

SECTION 3

Travancore and Orissa 81

WALTRAUD ERNST

5 **Medical developments and Western psychiatry in**
Travancore and Orissa 83

Introduction 83
A 'modern' and 'ideal' Indian state: Travancore 84
    Late nineteenth-century medical reforms and social
      stratification 87
Medical reforms and funding priorities 92
    The role of missionaries and caste reform 94
Religious welfare institutions and Brahmin privileges 96
Indigenous medicine and Vaidyasalas 99
Medical provision, government spending, and caste
in the twentieth century 103
    Gender 107

The lunatic asylum at Trivandrum during the late
  nineteenth century 109
Institutional statistics and reports 117
Psychiatric provision at Trivandrum in the early
  twentieth century 119
Formal classification and treatment of patients 125
Institutional trends and statistics 128
The Orissan states – "something rotten somewhere" 133
Conclusion 142

Index   160

Figures

5.1 Assigned religious affiliation of in- and out-patients treated
in Western government-sponsored institutions, in percentage,
1935/6 and 1945/6   105
5.2 Number of patients present at beginning of year; admitted,
discharged, and died during the year; total treated and
remaining at the end of the year, 1870/1 and 1946/7   129
5.3 Percentage of patients who died, of total number treated
during the year, 1870–1947   130
5.4 Percentage of patients remaining at the end of the year,
of total number treated, 1870–1947   131
5.5 Percentage of patients discharged, of total number treated
during the year, 1870–1947   132
5.6 Percentage of patients who died, of total number treated
during the year, with trendline, 1897–1947   155
5.7 Number of patients admitted, 1897–1947   156

Tables

1.1	Number of cases and deaths from plague in Mysore during the official year 1898–1899 (district and month-wise)	17
1.2	Number of inoculations from September 1898 to June 1899, Mysore	18
1.3	Quinquennial averages of mortality from plague, 1898–1899 to 1922–1923, Mysore	23
2.1	Growth of medical institutions in Mysore, 1881–1923	29
2.2	Pay scales of surgeons, 1918	30
2.3	Mortality and causes of death in Mysore, 1895–1900	34
3.1	Total number of lepers (1871)	47
4.1	Statement showing the operation of vaccination in the hill tracts of Ganjam for the years 1882–1887	66
4.2	Number of vaccinations and re-vaccinations for the years 1906–1940	67
4.3	Smallpox-related work done in the 'native' states under the supervision of the political agent (1906–1919)	69
5.1	Charity Hospital. Caste of patients treated, 1870/1	89
5.2	Civil Hospital. Caste of patients treated, 1870/1	90
5.3	Charges for medical department, 1870/1	93
5.4	Expenditure for 1870/71. Dewan's Report on the Finances, 10.11.1871	93
5.5	Applications for medical registrations, 1946/7	102
5.6	Attendance of in-patients and out-patients, in percentages, classified according to sexes, 1935/6 and 1945/6	107
5.7	Class and sex of the patients admitted during the year 1122 [1946/7]	108
5.8	Class and sex of the patients admitted during the year 1122 [1946/7]	109
5.9	The following return will show the number of patients admitted, the nature of the cases treated and the results. 1870/1	111
5.10	Number of 'insane' persons per 10,000 of the population, 1901	118
5.11	Number of 'insane' persons per 10,000 of population, by sex, 1901	119
5.12	Types of mental diseases in the mental hospital during the year 1120 [1944/5]	126
5.13	Therapy work in the Travancore Mental Hospital: electrical, by sex and outcome, 1946/7	128
5.14	Therapy work in the Travancore Mental Hospital: light treatment, by sex, 1946/7	128

About the authors

Waltraud Ernst is Professor in the History of Medicine at Oxford Brookes University, UK. Her research focuses on the history of mental illness in South Asia and her publications include *Mad Tales from the Raj* (1991; 2010) and *Colonialism and Transnational Psychiatry* (2013). She is the editor of *Work, Psychiatry and Society* (2016), *Transnational Psychiatry* (2010; with T. Mueller), *Crossing Colonial Historiographies* (2010; with A. Digby and P.B. Mukharji), *India's Princely States* (2007; with B. Pati), *The Normal and the Abnormal* (2006), *Plural Medicine, Tradition and Modernity* (2002), and *Race, Science and Medicine* (1999; with B.J. Harris).

Biswamoy Pati is a historian and teaches at the Department of History, Delhi University. His research is on the diversities of colonial and post-colonial India. At present he is attached to the Nehru Memorial Museum and Library, New Delhi, where he is researching on the Social Exclusion of the Adivasis and Outcastes/Dalits in colonial Orissa.

T.V. Sekher is Professor with Department of Population Policies and Programs at International Institute for Population Sciences (IIPS), Deemed University, Mumbai. A trained demographer, he researches on issues related to health, gender, and ageing in contemporary India, as well as on the history of population and public health in Princely Mysore. He is presently Fulbright-Nehru Academic and Professional Excellence Fellow at Cornell University, USA (2016–2017).

Acknowledgements

We are grateful to the Wellcome Trust for funding our project on 'Colonial Medicine and Indigenous Health Practices in Southern and Eastern Princely States of India, c. 1880–1960', which made research for this book possible. Participants at the conference on 'Health and Medicine in Indian Princely States', held at New Delhi in August 2011 and in particular Professor Barbara Ramusack, helped focus our attention on the complex social and political developments in the different states. Thanks are due to the staff at the archives visited during the course of our research, namely Karnataka State Archives Bangalore; Divisional Archives, Mysore; Libraries of Vidhan Soudha, ISEC, Mythic Society and Gokhale Institute of Public Affairs at Bangalore; Orissa State Archives, Bhubaneshwar; Kerala State Archives Thiruvananthapuram; Kerala Council for Historical Research Library and Resource Centre Thiruvananthapuram; National Archives New Delhi; Nehru Memorial Museum and Archives New Delhi; National Library of India Kolkata; India Office Records London; and Wellcome Library London.

T.V. Sekher is grateful to the late Professor P.N. Mari Bhat, the ex-Director of IIPS, and Professor G.K. Kadekodi, former Director of ISEC, for encouraging him to take up this study. He acknowledges fruitful discussions with Professor Tim Dyson, Professor Sanjoy Bhattacharya and Dr Saseendran Pallikadavath. He is thankful to Dr Naveen Thomas and Ms Preethi Bhat for research assistance at Bangalore and Mysore.

Biswamoy Pati would like to thank Mr Manmohan Krishna, whose research is on the social history of leprosy in colonial Bihar and Chotanagpur for his help.

Waltraud Ernst thanks Swati Chatterjee, Shilpi Rajpal and Dr Naveen Thomas for invaluable research assistance rendered in Kolkata, New Delhi and Bangalore respectively, and Professor Projit Mukharji and Dr Burton Cleetus for putting her in touch with colleagues in Thiruvananthapuram and Kozhikode.

We would also like to thank our publishers, and especially Lily Brown, for their patience.

Introduction

*Waltraud Ernst, Biswamoy Pati,
and T.V. Sekher*

Since the late 1980s the history and place of Western medicine in various colonial settings and in non-Western societies has been under scrutiny. Many intriguing questions have been raised concerning the role of medicine as a 'tool of empire' or 'water-carrier of colonialism'. These studies have contributed much to our understanding of the history of Western medicine in colonial South Asia. By focusing their analyses almost exclusively on the areas rendered 'pink' on the contemporary maps of empire on the Indian Subcontinent, namely on 'British India', the derived insights fail to consider that about two-fifths of the region were administered, more or less, by Indian agency. Although these Indian rulers may have recognized British suzerainty and, in some cases, were mere puppets in the hands of British officials, they were still ultimately responsible for the internal management of their states. Studies on medical systems in colonial India that focus exclusively on areas directly ruled by the British are bound to provide an incomplete picture of the political realities and medical developments on the Indian Subcontinent during the age of British imperialism. An in-depth assessment of medicine in 'Indian India', even if Indian ruled only in name, is essential to put previous findings on the nature and impact of 'colonial medicine' as it is conventionally called into broader perspective.

This book aims to contribute a new critical dimension to current debates on the meanings of 'colonial medicine'. It explores to what extent the development of Western-style medicine in the various Princely states can be characterized as 'colonial' – and, if so, what it is that makes it so. How were the changing paradigms and policies of an increasingly 'science-based' Western medicine implemented and received within the context of Princely India? Were they subject to modification and adaptation, and did they unfold in ways similar to those prevalent in the various presidencies or provinces of British India?

Given the fact that the British colonial power exerted indirect rule over Indian states, an important issue relates to the role of medicine as a means of justifying British overlordship in states dominated by rulers of diverse backgrounds and political inclinations. Most importantly though, how did Western medicine sit alongside other means of legitimation of Princely rule itself in the different states and which strata of indigenous society considered Western medicine as a social good that a state ought to provide? Issues of hegemony and its legitimation arise not only in relation to the supreme colonial power, but also in regard to the internal administration of individual states by a royal elite and its sycophants. And, last but not least, Indian rulers' ambition to please their overlords by implementing what was seen to be modern and enlightened policies, in order to avoid interference in internal affairs or even invasion, needs to be considered.

The book provides the basis for comparison between medicine in areas ruled indirectly by the British, in contrast to regions that were fully subjugated to Western colonial hegemony. Emphasis is on the extent to which the wider context of political governance and the cultural provenance of its agents had an impact on how medical measures were framed. In other words, was the provision of medical services dependent on whether Indians were ruled by British or indigenous political agency, and can distinctly different entities, such as a 'colonial psychiatry' in British India and an 'indigenous Western medicine' in Princely India, be identified? Given the diversity of Indian states, it is important to consider how any perceived backwardness or progressiveness of particular Indian areas impacted on the provision of Western medicine. It will be shown that there was as much variety in the quality and nature of Western medical provision in Princely states as there was in British India.

The authors map developments in public health (i.e. clean water supply, plague and smallpox prevention), the emergence of specialized medical institutions (leper and lunatic asylums), and the influence of Western medicine on indigenous medical communities (and their patients). The southern states of Mysore and Travancore and six of the 24 Orissa Princely states (Dhenkanal, Keonjhar, Mayurbhanj, Gangpur, Kalahandi, Nilgiri) will be at the centre of investigation. The former were comparatively large states, which, together with one of the Orissan states, Mayurbhanj, were considered as 'progressive' and 'enlightened'. The eastern tributary states of Orissa were small states; most of them were commonly described as 'backward' and 'despotic'.

The authors show that some of the selected states maintained strong links not only with British and British Indian medical practitioners and medical institutions, but also with eminent colleagues and organizations in Germany, France, and the United States. This provides new insights into the interplay of local adaptations of British medical approaches and policies with global exchanges between different national schools of thought in the formation of what is often vaguely, and all too simply, referred to as 'Western' or 'colonial' medicine. Neither Western nor colonial medicine was a monolith.

Diversity

Westerners are familiar with the colourful exotic representations of great Maharajas and Ranis and their ostentatious display of immense wealth. Images of Oriental princes that focus on their fabulous otherness have dominated public representations of Indian rulers. Exhibitions such as the one at the Victoria & Albert Museum in London in 2009 keep focusing on the aspects of splendour, luxury, and conspicuous consumption on the part of the ruling elite. How Princes' wealth was accrued – through the enslavement and exploitation of certain communities amongst their subject people – has elicited less attention. If matters of political, social, and economic governance figure at all in Western portrayals of Indian royalty, they tend to fluctuate between images of cruel despotism and cultural backwardness on the one hand and martial valour and enlightened attitudes on the other. Either way, socio-economic backwardness and progress are measured in terms of Western assumptions of modern governance. This is the case also in much of the post-colonial historiography, which tends to consider the former princes and their flunkies as conservative forces within the context of post-Independence political developments. However, given the great diversity of Indian states during the period of British rule, a more differentiated approach needs to be taken.

There were a little over 600 Princely states. They varied in size. Some were ruled by Hindu royalty, others by Muslims or Sikhs, with a population that did not always share its ruler's creed. Also referred to as 'Native States', these areas were projected as independent from the British, with various degrees of interference and control exercised over their administration, being 'advised', as it was euphemistically referred to, by British political 'residents' or diplomats. The laws that were in force in these enclaves were similar in some cases to those in force in British territories, but not necessarily so, and the inhabitants were not seen as British subjects. In fact, the 'native'-ruled states interacted with and were controlled and influenced by the supreme colonial power on the Subcontinent in many different ways.

It is important to keep in mind that the Princely states were highly diverse in terms of the social demographics of their population, their natural resources, and the cultural and personal preferences of their rulers. Mysore and Travancore exemplify states that were considered by the British and the Indian rulers themselves as 'enlightened' and 'progressive'. Their rulers encouraged features that appealed to the British, such as the exploitation of natural resources and encouragement of commerce and industry; development of infrastructure; and creation of the kind of social institutions (such as schools, hospitals, and municipal facilities) that were seen to be part and parcel of well-administered modern nation states in Western countries. In recognition of their progressive status – measured along Western lines – the British even granted to Mysore and Travancore during ceremonial occasions the highest and second highest number of gun salutes respectively that could be garnered by 'native' states. Such formal recognition by the supreme colonial power in South Asia was important to Indian rulers and subject of much jealousy between them. On the other end of the spectrum of Indian governance, there were states considered as 'backward' and even 'despotic'. Amongst them were some of the Orissa Princely or feudatory states, as they were referred to by the British. Together the Orissan states covered an area and population roughly equal to Ireland. Only some among them could boast any high ranks as far as gun salutes were concerned.

Mysore

Mysore was the second largest Princely state in India, extending over an area about the size of Scotland, with a population of about six million in 1911 and just over eight million in 1951. As in the case of a few other Indian Princely states, the 'progressive' image of Mysore is generally ascribed to administrative modernization, state support for social services, mainly for education and health, and the introduction of representative institutions.[1] For administrative purposes, Mysore state was divided into eight districts, each presided over by a deputy commissioner. Every district consisted of several *taluks* under the supervision of an *amildar*. The *amildar* was responsible for revenue administration and also for judicial and police work. The *taluk* was sub-divided into many *hoblis*, which were under the supervision of *sheikdars* or revenue officers.[2]

Princely Mysore had a well-organized Department of Public Health – partly due to the efforts of celebrated enlightened rulers and administrators, and partly due to the establishment of a well-structured administrative setup evolved during the 50 years of direct colonial rule. The British laid the foundation for a 'modern' administration in Mysore when they directly ruled the state from 1831 to 1881.[3] This period also witnessed the introduction of many new measures that gave a better outlook for the administrative machinery, with a high degree of functional specificity. Mysore was returned after half a century of British rule to the Wodeyar dynasty as a state with a 'good administration'.[4] A gradual transformation of administration resulted in the emergence of an administrative structure based upon the Madras and Bombay models. In that sense, the administration of Mysore can be considered as a 'child of colonialism'.[5] Mysore was called a 'model state' in view of the efficiency in the administration, benevolence of its rulers, and liberal political institutions. The Mysore Representative Assembly was created soon after the Maharaja's reinstatement in 1881. It had delegates from every *taluk*. At first, members were appointed by the government; in 1891 provision was made for election of members. The assembly held no power, but constituted a forum to air complaints against the government. However, its importance as a major contributor to Mysore's progressive reputation arises from the fact that, at its inception in 1881, it was the only representative institution of its size in the Subcontinent.[6] Some young princes from other native states were sent to Mysore to undergo administrative training because of its reputation as the best administered 'native' state in India.[7]

Mysore state had a well-established sanitation department. From the 1890s steps were taken to insure uniform policies with regard to epidemic control, vaccination, and development of sanitation facilities. This included legislation such as the Epidemic Diseases Regulation (1897), the Mysore Village Sanitary Regulation Act (1898), and the Vaccination Regulation Act of 1906. Along with the development of sanitary services, the government undertook the expansion of health services. In 1881, there were only 24 hospitals and dispensaries in the state, including two asylums, one for lunatics and the other for lepers. By 1918, the number of medical institutions increased to 178, and by 1923 to 200.[8] The establishment of rural health centres in 1931 was an important landmark in the provision of basic healthcare services. The activities of these centres included improvement of village sanitation, investigation and control of epidemics, immunization services, chlorination of drinking water sources, and the recording of births and deaths.

The establishment of many medical institutions – such as the leper asylum (1845), lunatic asylum (1848), Bowring and Lady Curzon Hospital (1866), K.R.

Hospital (1876), Maternity Hospital (1880), Medical School (1881), Marthas Hospital (1886), Epidemic Disease Hospital (1891), Vaccine Institute (1892), Public Health Institute (1895), Minto Eye Hospital (1896), and Victoria Hospital (1900) – constituted important steps in the development of health services in Mysore state.[9] Mysore also occupies a unique position in the history of family planning. The world's first government birth control clinics were established in Mysore City and in Bangalore as early as 1930, adding another dimension to the progressive measures in healthcare.[10]

Given this context, the Mysore chapters attempt to address the Princely administration of health and sanitation services and how it handled major crises such as the outbreak of plague in 1898. The gearing up of the entire administrative machinery to face this public health challenge was remarkable, with clear guidelines for the provision of relief and medical care and the allocation and utilization of funds. The presidents of municipalities were given the power to question and demand an enquiry into the cause of every death. However, the administration's plague-control measures clashed with popular values and cultural beliefs. In many places, the segregation of contacts and mandatory hospitalization of victims attracted strong opposition from the public and compulsory measures had to be abandoned. Members of the representative assembly took the Princely administration to task by fearlessly voicing people's concerns and questioning the government on relief measures, and specifically on ignoring the villages, during epidemics.

The Mysore chapters attempt to understand how far Western influence and British rule had an impact not only on medical practices, but also on health administration and sanitary reforms in a 'progressive' and 'enlightened' Princely state.

The states of Orissa

As a part of the Bengal presidency and, since 1936, as a province Orissa had as many as 26 Princely states. Out of these 24 merged with Orissa at the time of independence (between 1947 and 1949), with two of them (Kharswan and Singbhum) merging with Bihar. Geographically located in what was identified as the non-coastal, western interior, they were also referred to as *garhjats*. Whereas the coastal tract comprising Cuttack, Puri, and Balasore had been tapped for land revenue by the Mughals, the western interior had remained out of this process. In terms of size, Mayurbhanj was the largest Princely state (4,243 square miles) whereas Tigiria (46 square miles) was the smallest one. The Orissa chapters focus on Mayurbhanj, Keonjhar, Gangpur, Kalahandi, Nilgiri and Dhenkanal – six of Orissa's erstwhile Princely states. The choice of states has been dictated primarily on the basis of the availability of source materials, especially since most of the states did not publish materials related to the prevailing health system in a regular way. Nevertheless, as will be shown, the chosen six states provide a representative picture of health conditions related to leprosy and smallpox and help us understand the realities associated with health initiatives and policies that were introduced by the princes.

Following the annexation of Orissa by the British in 1805, the nineteenth century saw the Princely rulers being both invented and cradled by colonialism. This process included the implementation of land settlements – based on *sanads* or agreements – which sought to stabilize colonialism's access to resources, as well as the power and authority of the Princely rulers. An annual tribute or *peshkush* was paid to the British colonial government.[11] The colonial land revenue settlements were modelled along the lines of the 'permanent settlement', first introduced by the British in Bengal, Bihar, and Orissa in 1793. This meant that the princes had property rights over land. However, the cultivators had no land rights and the tax they had to pay to their chiefs was left undefined. Consequently, the colonial interventions had far-reaching implications for the Indian states, which were supposedly not under direct colonial control. The agrarian interventions reinforced the existing class/caste and gender hierarchies, even as they secured a stable supply of revenue.[12] In fact, this interactive aspect had several implications and influenced the health policies and initiatives undertaken by the Princely rulers.

In British-ruled areas, health matters remained focused on the colonial army in the early years. Nevertheless, with the end of the English East India Company and the 'Crown' taking over India (1858), gradual shifts were observable. This was primarily associated with ideas of introducing a system of governance and civil administration. In this context matters affecting the public, as well as public health, were taken up in terms of policies. These were more pronounced and visible in the directly administered 'temporarily settled' areas of Orissa than in the Princely states. Of course, we do not always have full documentation of the measures taken in the latter, as regular reports were lacking in regard to public health and the relationship with the colonial power still remained to be stabilized.

Enumeration and census operations initiated in the late 1870s contributed towards, amongst other features, polarizing identities and relationships. However, this pales into insignificance if compared with the land revenue settlements that were created by British colonialism. For example, the Mayurbhanj *darbar* paid Rs 1,001 as *peshkush*, though it had the largest income amongst the Orissan states, amounting to Rs 2,820,000 annually by the 1930s. The Dhenkanal state paid Rs 5,099 as *peshkush* for the colonial administration. The gross land rental of the state increased from Rs. 63,316 in 1846 to Rs 239,347 by 1923. The Talcher *darbar* had a treaty with the East India Company in 1848 and paid a *peshkush* of Rs 1,040, but its land revenue income increased from Rs 21,290 in 1846 to Rs. 58,971 in 1913. Similarly, the Nilgiri state's land revenue increased more than five times between 1853 and 1920, although the *darbar* paid a fixed *peshkush* of Rs 2,108 as per the agreement with the East India Company in 1809.[13] This meant that peasants and tribals lost out in two ways: they had no rights over lands (in fact even customary rights over forest, pastures, and rivers were progressively undermined over the nineteenth century itself) and they were left mercilessly to the whims of the *darbars* when it came to taxation demands, which increased steadily from the 1860s to the 1940s.[14] In other words, while the *darbars* were able to accumulate considerable resources, they did not elect to spend them on sectors such as health.

The question of legitimacy is important in regard to health interventions that occurred over the latter half of the nineteenth century. The princes and their *darbars* were associated with two contradictory processes. They went to great lengths to prove their 'ancientness' and invented *bansabalis* or chronicles of their ancestry to legitimize and validate their claims, while simultaneously flirting with 'modernity'. Both these features had a direct bearing on their *raison d'être* and mode of functioning. Thus, the former reflected the essentially conservative logic of their existence while modernity as espoused in British-ruled areas had a direct bearing on their health policies. In fact, it made the princes join the bandwagon of 'modernity' to legitimize their position in the eyes of the British and the emerging Indian middle class. In this sense, measures such as health policies served to legitimize colonialism.[15] And, seen from the point of view of colonialism, health policies adopted by the Princely rulers and their *darbars* demonstrated the success of its 'civilizing mission'. Consequently what needs to be stressed is that through the incorporation of the project of 'modernity' the *darbars* legitimized their existence as much as they legitimized colonialism. And, it is here that an area such as public health proved to be rather significant.

The Orissa chapters will therefore focus on how the Princely *darbars* conceptualized and related to public health. It is equally important to assess if the states' people, composed largely of poor *Adivasis* (or tribals) and outcastes had access to and benefited from any health-related initiatives, and to gauge how they survived in areas where these did not exist.

Travancore

Travancore joined the Indian Union late, in 1949, when it formed Travancore-Cochin, with the former Travancore ruler being installed as *rajpramukh*, or governor, and, finally, Kerala in 1956. Unlike Mysore, Travancore did not experience an interlude of direct British rule. It therefore lacked the kind of head start in terms of colonial administrative setup on which Mysore could construct its image as an 'enlightened' and well-governed state. Still, like its fellow model state, Travancore had a British resident who 'advised' its ruler and administration was closely linked with and subject to scrutiny by the British-ruled, neighbouring Madras presidency. The British resident ensured that matters of political administration, medical provision, and welfare provision were handled in accordance with Western blueprints and were at least broadly acceptable to British economic and political interests and Western social mores. Frederick Roberts (1832–1914), the famous 'Lord Roberts of Kandahar' who had 41 years of service in India, put the British position in a nutshell:

> Notwithstanding the high civilization, luxury, and refinement to be found in these Natives States, my visits to them strengthened my opinion that, however capable and enlightened the Ruler, he could have no chance of holding his country if deprived of the guiding hand of the British Government as embodied in the Resident.[16]

The extraordinarily degrading treatment of lower and outcastes in Travancore on the part of 'caste Hindus', sanctioned by royalty and the *darbar*, was frequently bemoaned by the British and vehemently condemned by missionaries. However, as in other regions, the wealth of the princes, and of the elite and religious groups that supported them, was based on the exploitation of those relegated to the bottom rungs of the social hierarchy. And as Roberts observed following his meeting with the ruler of Travancore in the 1880s, while "his appearance was distinguished, and his manners those of a well-bred, courteous English gentleman of the old school", he "dared not do anything without the sanction of the priests, and he spent enormous sums in propitiating them".[17] The abolition of enslavement and improvements of the condition of lower- and outcaste communities was eventually hard won, against rather than with, the support of the princes and the British who enshrined, as in the case of the Orissan states, prevalent power relations and repressive practices.

Echoing developments in regard to public health and education in British-ruled areas, an "extension of the means of medical aid in the country" was mooted and so-called "poverty schools" as well as a "higher branch of education" founded during the 1860s and 1870s. In regard to the former, emphasis was on the establishment of dispensaries and small hospitals, and provision of smallpox vaccination for military staff and workers connected with plantations and infrastructure projects such as dams and roads. Like in British India during the early nineteenth century, state medicine focused on areas that were strategically important for defence and internal security purposes respectively, and for economic development or exploitation of natural resources.

The 1890s were characterized by a continued focus on vaccination, malaria, and plague prevention; improvements of conservancy, mainly in conurbations; and the reorganization of the medical department and the collection of vital statistics.[18] The slow extension of medical and public health provision beyond urban areas began in the 1920s and 1930s, occasioned not least by pressure from vocal interest groups, members of the legislative council, and the local press.[19] The Village Sanitary Act, which emulated the measures taken in Mysore, was introduced in 1925 to remedy some of the problems but underfunding rendered it more or less ineffective. Public health did not figure highly amongst the spending priorities of the state. Provision for mental health, as will be shown in the Travancore chapter, figured even less so.

Conventional histories of the development of medicine and public health along modern lines attribute a major role to the Rockefeller Foundation, which was invited by the Travancore government in 1928 to advise on the reorganization of health-related services. Yet, local pressure groups were no less influential in pushing for greater accessibility to and extension of Western-style facilities. Still, consultation of American advisors highlights the important re-orientation towards expertise that existed beyond British colonial blueprints in some Indian states (and even in British-ruled provinces following the devolution of internal affairs from central government to the provinces). What is more, successive rulers and their *darbars* provided patronage also for indigenous approaches to healing, which had led to the formation and financial support of an Indian, alongside the Western, medical department from the late nineteenth century onwards. From this period, Travancore had also mooted employment of its own people in official positions rather than relying on staff sent by the government of Madras. This contributed to the emergence of a Travancorian middle class and weakened the umbilical cord that connected the state with the British-ruled Madras presidency.

By the 1940s, Travancore could boast a comparatively well-developed public health and medical system based on both Western and indigenous modes of healing, which had been complemented since the early nineteenth century by some excellent establishments run by missionaries. However, in terms of access to service provision, an urban and elite focus continued to prevail in particular in regard to Western facilities. Caste-based discrimination was challenged by caste reform and political movements from the late nineteenth century, but continued to be supported by some influential members of the royal household and their hangers-on.

The last section in this book focuses on developments in regard to mental health in Travancore. While the mental hospital at Mysore became a facility located at the cutting edge of Western psychiatric ideas and practices that attracted high-profile visitors from across the world and highly trained staff on account of well-established scientific networks and support by influential members of the urban elite, Travancore's facilities remained restricted in scope and vision. In the Orissan states, mental health provision along Western lines was more or less absent. Contempt for and prejudice against tribal people (or Adivasis), who made up a substantial proportion of the population in these states, were shared by Indian rulers and their *darbars* as well as by the British. The latter tended to put semi-nomadic peoples at the bottom rungs of the racial hierarchy, criminalized them, and forced them to become sedentary, lest they could cut across the clear lines of regional boundaries and what was supposed to be permanent settlements for taxation purposes. The former exploited them woefully, as the Orissan chapters will show. The numerically relatively insignificant urban elites were able to access mental health provision in neighbouring British areas, while tribals fell back on their own cultural modes of dealing with mental conditions.

Neither British nor Princely interests were jeopardized by inadequate or lack of Western-style mental health care provision. In any case, the 'civilizing mission' was selective in its remit, being based on existing blueprints and developments in the colonial motherland. There, too, healthcare was not freely available to all. In our assessment of health provision in British colonies and in indirectly ruled areas, we need to keep in mind that the majority of people in Britain itself did not benefit from access to medical treatment until the formation under a Labour government of the National Health Service in 1948.

Notes

1 For details see, Barbara Ramusack, *The Indian Princes and Their States*, Cambridge: Cambridge University Press, 2004.
2 For details see, James Manor, *Political Change in an Indian State: Mysore 1917–1955*, Delhi: Manohar Publications, 1977.
3 C. Hayavadana Rao, *Mysore Gazetteers, Compiled for Government*, various volumes, Bangalore: Government Press, 1927–1930.
4 Rao, *Mysore Gazetteers*.
5 Bjorn Hettne, *The Political Economy of Indirect Rule: Mysore 1881–1947*, New Delhi: Ambika Publications, 1978.

6   Along with the Representative Assembly, another representative political institution, the Legislative Council, with limited powers to vote on proposed legislation, was created in 1907. However, the Council contained majority of government officials and nominees. For details see: Manor, *Political Change*.

7   M.M. Ismail, *My Public Life, Recollections and Reflections of Sir Mirza Ismail*, London, 1954, and Manor, *Political Change*.

8   C. Hayavadana Rao, *Mysore Gazetteers*, Vol. 4 (Administrative).

9   *Ibid.*

10 P.H. Rayappa and T.V. Sekher, 'Administration of Health Services in Karnataka', in S. Ramanathan (ed.), *Landmarks in Karnataka Administration* (pp. 316–341), New Delhi: Indian Institute of Public Administration and Uppal Publishers, 1998.

11 For details see Ranajit Guha, *A Rule of Property for Bengal: An Essay on the Idea of Permanent Settlement*, Paris: Mouton, 1963; Dharma Kumar (ed.), *The Cambridge Economic History of India, vol. II, c. 1757–1970*, Hyderabad: Orient Longman, 1984, especially pp. 86–177.

12 For details see Biswamoy Pati, 'The Order of Legitimacy: Princely Orissa, 1850–1947', in Waltraud Ernst and Biswamoy Pati (eds.), *India's Princely States: People, Princes and Colonialism*, Oxford: Routledge, 2007, 86–7 (85–98).

13 For details see Nilamani Senapati and Nabin K. Sahu (eds.), *Orissa District Gazetteers: Mayurbhanj*, Cuttack: Orissa Government Press, 1967, 72–5; *Memoranda on the Indian States, 1932*, Delhi: Government of India, 1933, 222–3, puts the average annual revenue at Rs 28,20,000 and the payment to the government was Rs 1,068, an increase of Rs 67 over what was paid in 1812; *Final Report on the Settlement of the Dhenkanal Feuda-tory State Orissa 1923–4*, vol. I, Berhampur: Board of Revenue, Orissa, 1966, 26–9, 40; *The Memoranda on the Indian States 1930*, Calcutta: Central Publication Branch, Government of India, 1931, 222–3, gives us the figures of the *peshkush*; *Report on the Land Revenue Settlement 1911–1912, Talcher State*, Cuttack: Board of Revenue, 1963, 33; and *Final Report on the Nilgiri Settlement 1917–22*, Berhampur: Sarada Press, no date, 1, 41; as mentioned, the land revenue increased five-fold between 1853 and 1922.

14 For details see, H.K. Mahtab, Lalmohan Pattnaik and Balvantrai Mehta (eds.), *Report of the Enquiry Committee: Orissa States*, Cuttack: Orissa Mission Press, 1939; R.K. Ramadhyani, *Report on the Land Tenures and the Revenue System of the Orissa and Chattisgarh States, vol. III, the Individual States*, Berhampur: Indian Law Publications, 1942.

15 Pati, 'The Order of Legitimacy', 94–5.

16 Frederick Roberts, *Forty-one Years in India: From Subaltern to Commander-in-Chief*, London: MacMillan, 1898, 502.

17 Roberts, *Forty-one Years*, 502.

18 Kerala State Archives, Thiruvananthapuram, 1896, Cover File, 7155.

19 Joel T. Wins, *A History of Health and Family Welfare Department in Kerala*, University of Kerala, PhD Dissertation, 2013, Chapter 1, 46.

Section 1

Mysore

T.V. Sekher

1 Plague administration in Princely Mysore

Resistance, riots, and reconciliation

In the early twentieth century, one of India's most feared and deadliest diseases was the plague. Plague ravaged India for two decades and sporadically thereafter, from its first appearance in Bombay city in August 1896, leading to the death of at least 12 million people.[1] India was recorded as having suffered about 95 percent of the world's plague mortality during the period 1894 to 1938.[2] The population pressure, crowding, malnutrition, and lack of sanitation increased the vulnerabilities of the population to plague infection. It is also argued that apart from inducing massive mortality, the epidemic greatly disrupted millions of people – forced to evacuate their homes, stay in temporary sheds (camps), and detained for observations. "Plague was a savage cause of death and, equally, of social turmoil between the state and populace" (p-723).[3] The approach of the colonial rulers, especially imposed during the plague epidemic of 1896–1897, provoked extremely hostile public reaction and stirred "up a great tide of alienation from Western medicine" (p-237), which in course of time forced the state to retreat to a less interventionist policy.[4]

In Mysore Province, with a population of 4,943,604 as per the Census of 1891,[5] the plague first appeared in Bangalore on 12 August 1898. The epidemic wreaked havoc, particularly in Bangalore City and neighbouring areas. From 1898 to 1923, the disease claimed 2,05, 422 victims in the state.[6] The outbreak of plague in Bombay (now Mumbai) in 1896 gave rise to anxiety for both administration and public, particularly in the adjoining states. By the end of the year 1897, the plague had established itself and was increasing in virulence at Hubli, a populous town on the direct line of railway communication with Bangalore and only 80 miles from the Mysore frontier. This circumstance deepened the public anxiety and it was recognized that all possible precautions should be taken to prevent the introduction of the disease into the state.

While addressing the *Dasara* Session of the Mysore Representative Assembly on 17 October 1899, the Dewan, K.Seshadri Iyer, stated:

> It was on 12 August, 1898, and in the city of Bangalore, that the plague first made its appearance in the State. The exact manner in which the disease was conveyed to Bangalore has not been satisfactorily traced, though there is a good ground for believing that its importation was in some way due to its prevalence in an epidemic form at Hubli and other stations on the

Southern-Mahratta Railway, among whose coolies it first occurred, and to the families and friends of whose employees it was for sometime confined before spreading first to localities in close proximity to the railway goods-shed at Bangalore, and then to the other parts of the city. When the disease once gained a foothold in the Bangalore city, it soon spread with increasing virulence in every direction, passing rapidly into the Civil and Military stations, and the rest of the Bangalore district, and then into the Mysore city and the Mysore and Kolar districts and parts of the Tumkur district. The only districts that were altogether free of indigenous cases were Shimoga, Hassan, Kadur, and Chitaldrug.[7]

Administrative measures to control plague

During the earlier years of the epidemic, the preventive measures were mostly aimed at the destruction of the pathogenic-microorganisms, the *plague bacillus*, which was supposed to be the independent causative agent in the transmission of the disease. When the bubonic plague broke out in the neighbouring Dharwar district[8] (part of Bombay Presidency) on 17 October 1897, the Mysore administration was alerted and took certain precautionary measures such as examination of passengers coming into Bangalore by rail and road, establishment of a plague hospital, and segregation of population and setting up of health camps. The government passed the Mysore Epidemic Diseases Regulation Act in 1897, which granted extensive powers to the government to deal with the plague. The Epidemic Diseases Hospital at Bangalore (originally known as *Chattram* Hospital), started in 1891 and located at a safe distance from the Railway Station, was available for accommodation and treatment of cases of infectious and communicable diseases amongst the residents and the pilgrims and others arriving by train. The government also issued a notification, dated 10 February 1898, by which the Presidents of the Municipalities were given power to question and to demand an enquiry into the cause of every death:

> The President of the Municipality was empowered to require that the certificate of a medical officer should be obtained, showing the cause of every death within two hours after such death, and to presume, if a burial or cremation took place without such a certificate, that the death was due to plague. The rule was brought into force on 1 January, 1899, in Bangalore.[9]

Another important development was the passage of the Village Sanitation Regulation in 1898, to regulate conservancy measures in villages.

Some of the important precautionary measures initiated by the Princely Administration in Mysore[10] were:

(i) The establishment of railway medical inspection stations, at Harihar, Yeswantpur, Bowringpet, Bangalore Cantonment, Kengeri and Mysore City, under Notifications of the Resident or of the Durbar.

(ii)   The establishment of outposts and road inspection stations, manned by Police and village servants and within easy reach of segregation sheds; also of frontier inspection stations, especially in the Chitaldrug and Shimoga borders, systematically patrolled by special Inspectors; and the watching of the Bangalore City and Kolar Gold Fields at all approaches.

(iii) The examination of passengers by rail and road.

(iv)   The detention, observation, or escort to their destination of persons arriving from infected areas or suspected of carrying infection.

(v)   The disinfection of houses and of passengers.

(vi)   The imposition on householders and others of the obligation to give immediate information of the occurrence of plague cases.

(vii) The introduction of the "supervision system" into the Bangalore City, which was divided for the purpose into circles under Superintendents and further subdivided into blocks under Supervisors, who made daily inspection of each house with a view to ascertain all arrivals, departures, sicknesses, and deaths. On the outbreak of plague, this system was replaced by the Ward system, the Cities of Bangalore and Mysore being divided into Wards under Civil Ward Officers assisted by Medical Officers.

(viii) The establishment of temporary plague hospitals and segregation and health camps at centres most likely to become affected.

(ix)   The stationing of Police constables at each burial and cremation ground in the Bangalore City to register every funeral, and, as far as possible, to ascertain the cause of death.

(x)   The encouragement of the destruction of rats by offer of rewards and otherwise.

(xi)   The prohibition of fairs and festivals at which large crowds were likely to collect, or of the attendance threat of persons from infected areas.

(xii) The distribution of leaflets and the holding of meetings for explaining to the people the dangers of plague, the object of the measures adopted by government, and the necessity for popular co-operation.

(xiii) The enforcement of special sanitary improvements in towns and villages.

The plague prevention measures reflected the seriousness of the Mysore government to address the epidemic, which had already set in the neighbouring Bombay Presidency.[11] For the prompt and effective administration of preventive measures, V.P. Madhava Rao, the Inspector General of Police at that time, was placed in charge of the measures with extensive discretionary powers, along with the Senior Surgeon and Sanitary Commissioner. On his elevation to the Council in April 1898, Madhava Rao continued to be in charge of the precautionary measures, under the designation of 'Plague Commissioner in Mysore'.[12] Even before the outbreak of plague in the province, the preventive measures cost Rs. 29, 495 from Provincial Funds, and Rs. 15,859 from Municipal Funds, during the year 1897–1898.[13]

In October 1898, a separate temporary department, the 'Plague Department', was set up as a branch of the General Department of the government. The plague operations in the Bangalore City were at first under the control of the President of the Municipality aided by the Ward Officers, but as plague increased, a Chief Plague Officer was appointed in October 1898. In the Mysore City these operations were under the control of the Deputy Commissioner, assisted by a Chief Plague Officer and Ward Officers. In other places they were directed by the Deputy Commissioners assisted by the Superintendents of Police. In the Bangalore and Mysore Districts, there were separate District Plague Officers. In the Tumkur and Kolar Districts, the Police Superintendents were themselves District Plague Officers; a Special Plague Officer was appointed temporarily for the Kolar Gold Fields. In the other districts, no extra officers were specially appointed for plague duty, but the Assistant Commissioners, *Amildars*,[14] and Hospital Assistants gave assistance in addition to their own duties.[15]

In spite of the precautions adopted, with a focus on Bangalore City, the plague made its way into the city in August 1898, the first case occurring on the 12th of that month. For the first four weeks (i.e. up to 9 September 1898), cases were few and they occurred at intervals of a day or two. But from 9 September, the mortality rose. In October, the plague became an epidemic in Bangalore City, with 1,393 new cases for the month of October and the total mortality went up to 2,807. Up to 9 November 1898, the disease went on increasing, in terms of the number of cases, deaths, and the extent of area affected. Altogether, there were 14,831 attacks and 12,272 deaths from plague in the Mysore State during the year 1898–1899. Bangalore City alone recorded 3346 attacks and 2665 deaths, and in Mysore City, 2667 attacks and 2171 deaths were recorded.[16] The estimated plague mortality was probably 75 per 1000 in Bangalore City, and 35 per thousand in Mysore City during the period of August 1898 to March 1899 (p-1095).[17] Table 1.1 presents the district-wise details of plague incidences in Mysore State, indicating 83 percent of those infected with plague did not survive, and showing a plague mortality of 2.53 per 1000 population as state average in the first year of the epidemic. This figure for Bangalore district was as high as ten per 1000 population.[18]

Did the hospitalization help in reducing plague mortality? As per records, amongst the 2938 hospitalized cases, 1973 deaths were reported in the first year of the outbreak (1898–1899). Sixty-seven percent of the infected inmates in the five hospitals/plague camps did not survive.[19] Considering that the province was witness to high incidence of plague deaths, as shown in Table 1.1, the mortality of hospitalized cases was comparatively less. This might have prompted the authorities to take measures for mandatory hospitalization of infected persons.

With the virulence of the epidemic spreading, the Government initiated measures for prevention and suppression. Briefly, the measures can be summarized as given below[20]:

(i)   All passengers from infected areas, by rail or by road, were examined and placed under observation. Disinfection arrangements were made at the Bangalore and Mysore City Railway Stations.

(ii) People living in infected localities were asked to vacate.

Table 1.1 Number of cases and deaths from plague in Mysore during the official year 1898–1899 (district and month-wise)

Districts	July		August		September		October		November		December		January		February		March		April		May		June		Total		Percent of deaths to total cases	Ratio of deaths per 1000 population
	Cases	Deaths	Cases	Deaths	Cases	Deaths	Cases	Deaths	Cases	Deaths	Cases	Deaths	Cases	Deaths	Cases	Deaths	Cases	Deaths	Cases	Deaths	Cases	Deaths	Cases	Deaths	Cases	Deaths		
Bangalore	–	–	22	15	234	145	1513	1196	1604	1313	1998	1770	2073	1924	550	497	191	164	33	33	37	28	83	52	8338	7137	85.60	10.15
Kolar	–	–	–	–	2	2	53	39	88	67	267	216	610	520	273	247	315	226	260	192	195	128	100	69	2163	1706	78.87	2.89
Tumkur	–	–	–	–	2	2	20	15	136	99	404	293	288	216	89	84	44	32	5	4	–	–	–	–	988	745	75.41	1.28
Mysore	–	–	–	–	2	2	18	12	67	66	105	73	862	650	1239	1003	548	479	175	156	153	108	158	125	3327	2674	80.37	2.26
Hassan	–	–	–	–	–	–	1	1	1	–	–	–	–	–	–	–	–	–	–	–	–	–	–	–	2	1	50.00	0.00
Shimoga	–	–	–	–	–	–	–	–	–	–	–	–	–	–	–	–	–	–	–	–	–	–	–	–	–	–	–	–
Kadur	–	–	–	–	–	–	4	4	1	1	1	–	–	–	–	–	–	–	–	–	–	–	–	–	6	5	83.33	0.02
Chitaldrug	–	–	–	–	–	–	4	3	2	1	1	–	–	–	–	–	–	–	–	–	–	–	–	–	7	4	57.14	0.00
Total	–	–	22	15	240	151	1613	1270	1899	1547	2776	2352	3833	3310	2151	1831	1098	901	473	385	385	264	341	246	14831	12272	82.75	2.53

Source: Annual Medical and Sanitary Report of Mysore, 1898–1899, General and Revenue Department, Government of Mysore, Karnataka State Archives, p-16.

(iii) Infected houses and infected persons were subjected to systematic disinfection. In rural areas, un-roofing of thatched houses and their exposure to sun and air, as well as lime washing of houses, was adopted. Chemical disinfection was mostly confined to the larger towns.

(iv) Compulsory segregation was resorted to for some time, but was found to be extremely unpopular and ineffective, besides being very costly and difficult to enforce.[21]

(v) Accommodation was provided in camps for contacts and persons living in infected areas. Numerous camps were established for the accommodation of the healthy who wished to quit infected localities. In many cases, especially away from the larger towns, the people preferred to make sheds of their own. Free timber and bamboos were provided to the poorest classes to enable them to make their own sheds.

(vii) Relief works for the indigent were started wherever necessary.

(viii) Every encouragement was given for inoculation. The status of inoculations in the first year of the plague outbreak (up to 30 June 1899) is detailed in Table 1.2.

(ix) Provision was made in Government Plague Hospitals for the treatment of the sick. No specific or particular line of treatment was adopted and each case was treated on its own merits.[22]

Table 1.2 Number of inoculations from September 1898 to June 1899, Mysore

Districts/city	Total number of persons inoculated	Attacks amongst the inoculated	Deaths amongst the inoculated
Bangalore City	36,259	236	120
Bangalore District	9,456	91	29
Mysore City	29.993	174	123
Mysore District	1,793	13	10
Kolar District (excluding the Kolar Gold Fields)	6,200	19	5
Kolar Gold Fields	11,619	38	24
Tumkur Town	2,071	97	86
Tumkur District (excluding Tumkur Town)	1,238	22	8
Chitaldrug District	66	–	–
Kadur District	444	–	–
Hassan District	325	–	–
Shimoga District	270	–	–

Source: Report of the Administration of Mysore for the Four Years 1895–96 to 1898–99, p-62, Karnataka State Archives, Bangalore.

(x)   Arrangements were made for the accurate registration of deaths and a system of death certificates was introduced in the Bangalore and Mysore Cities.

(xi)   A large number of houses condemned as unfit for habitation were demolished in Bangalore and Mysore Cities, and also in the other infected localities, and the congested areas were opened out by the construction of roads, streets, and lanes.

(xii)   Two large extensions covering an area of 731 acres (the Southern or Basavanagudi Extension covering 440 acres; and the Northern or Malleswaram Extension, covering 291 acres), and capable of providing accommodation for over 20,000 persons, were laid out in Bangalore City. Sites were marked out and assigned amongst the different communities, and several houses were constructed.

(xiii) Advances of a year's pay were sanctioned to government servants who desired to build houses in the any one of the above extensions of Bangalore City. Advances of three months' pay were also sanctioned in certain infected localities to enable government servants to put up sheds.

(xiv)   Special attention was paid to sanitation both in cities and in villages.

(xv)   Additional establishments of nurses, doctors, servants, Police constables, ambulance staff, transport and disinfection staff, etc., were appointed for the efficient carrying out of anti-plague measures.

The prevention and suppression measures against plague outbreak was supported through generous financial allocations. In fact, the financial statement of the Mysore government showed a deficit of Rs. 20,43,307 in the year 1898–1899, of which there was an "exceptional expenditure" for plague administration to the tune of Rs. 7,39,406.[23] The major share of this was used in the two cities of Bangalore (Rs. 2,93,210) and Mysore (Rs 1,10,230). Two major heads of the expenditures were the erection of sheds for contacts and health camps (20 percent) and for additional police (15 percent).

Public resistance

The administration took strong initiatives for prompt evacuation, encouraged exterminating rodents, published methods of proper sanitation and ventilation, and even assigned cash rewards for taking such measures. The system of destroying rats was encouraged by the payment of rewards. For every rat killed, one *anna* was offered as cash incentive. The importance of rat destruction as a plague preventive measure had been impressed upon the people and they were asked to keep their houses free from dangerous rodents. In villages, people were moved out of their houses; but in towns the people were generally averse to a relocation, mainly because of the difficulty of ensuring the safety of their property. People were allowed to deposit their valuables in public treasuries during the period of evacuation. Police protection was afforded to them during their stay in camps. Inoculation was introduced in September 1898, and teachers were instructed to ensure that all school children were inoculated. Directions were issued to heads of institutions to refuse admission if any student failed to comply with this rule. Rewards were also paid at the rate of four *annas* for each adult and two *annas* for each child inoculated from the labour classes. Through a local ballad (*lavani*), the message of hygiene was used to spread amongst the students and public. *Jatras* (public gatherings during temple festivals) were prohibited. Most of these anti-plague measures did not go down well with the sentiments of the public.

Like in other parts of the country, the inoculation and Western medicines were opposed by the local people. This opposition was more evident when there was segregated hospitalization. As Madhava Rao writes, "the patients preferred to be left alone without any treatment and in some cases they had recourse to indigenous drugs".[24] Both hospitalization and segregation were opposed, also fearing the violation of caste rules. In fact, measures of the administration to tackle the epidemic were perceived to be against the socio-religious sentiments of the locals. In the bordering Kannada-speaking district of Dharwar, the suicide of a Brahmin priest, Hayagrivacharya,[25] further catapulted the public resentment against the anti-plague measures of the administration.[26] Muslims also strongly opposed the measures of the administration to move the sick to hospitals and camps. In some places, separate *gosha* accommodations were provided to *burkha*-clad Muslim women.[27] According to a report from the Deputy Commissioner of Bangalore District, there were many instances wherein the plague victims were buried hurriedly and secretly, and even disfigured the face of the dead bodies to prevent identification and bundled them up in mats or *kumblis* and threw the corpses into gutters and drains, or left the plague patients in a hapless condition and fled to avoid the plague.[28]

The hospitals and camps were looked upon as jails and slaughterhouses by many. The administrations' efforts to purify the drinking water was interpreted by people as an attempt to poison them, and resulted in people not using the public water taps. As an expression of their hostility towards the administrative measures to curtail plague, the public set on fire some plague sheds. The Health Officer of Bangalore City, Achut Rao, was at the receiving end of the public ire, "had stones pelted at him by youth who disapproved of inoculation".[29] As argued by Gustafson, "[For the masses], inoculation caused leprosy, madness, and impotence."[30] In fact, the effort to inoculate people against plague even affected the regular vaccination work in the Province.[31]

When the relief measures were at its peak, the Municipal Administration had to face many other challenges. Employees of the Municipality stopped work, demanding higher wages. The Municipal Administration also had difficulty in inducing conservancy workers to clear the dead bodies thrown into gutters. It was forced to engage bullock carts. The situation became more grave and complicated as the plague became more virulent, the conservancy workers refusing to work.

Public resentment was echoed in many vernacular newspapers such as *Karnataka Prakasika* and *Vrittanta Chintamani*. These reports openly criticized the measures and actions of the government to control the epidemic.[32] These reports further fuelled the existing public resentment. The administration had to resort to use of force to control hostile crowds. One such incident near Srirangapatam, in November 1898, became known as the 'Ganjam Riots', a historic event in the people's agitations against anti-plague measure of the Mysore *Durbar*.

Plague and riots: the Ganjam case

Ganjam or *Shahar Ganjam*, a predominantly agricultural village, was a suburb of the Srirangapatam. It also had a number of well-to-do merchant residents engaged in cloth business.[33] Three weavers from Bangalore came to Ganjam on 2 November 1898. Two of them were infected with plague and one died on 6 November 1898. The second patient died on 10 November 1898. The corpse of the first victim was cremated without much opposition and the authorities were able to disinfect the shed. However, in the case of the second death, locals refused the cremation of the body, apprehending that the victim had been poisoned. People resisted and pelted stones at the officers who had come to cremate the body. The Plague Commissioner, V.P. Madhava Rao, assisted by the police, inspected the area and succeeded in restoring order. But the government efforts to arrest the rioters did not succeed owing to the angry protesters. However, after eight days, on 18 November, a large contingent of police with full emergency powers raided the village and arrested 55 persons suspected to be behind the riots and violence. Locals from Ganjam and neighbouring areas retaliated with sticks, swords, and guns, and tried to rescue the arrested persons. The police had to open fire to control the agitating mob, resulting in death and injury to some villagers.[34]

Although the Ganjam riots were brought under control, it marked a turning point in the plague administration in Mysore State. Government realized that, to implement its plague-control measures, it needed the support of the people. This was possible only through persuasion and taking the people into confidence about the threats from the epidemic and the measures to tackle it. This change in government strategy was seen in the notification issued on 1 December 1898 abolishing compulsory segregation. For instance, after the re-appearance of plague in Bangalore City towards the latter part of June 1899, the abolition of compulsory segregation was resolved upon for that place and assurance was given in a Notification that

> neither patients nor contacts will be removed to hospital or camp against their will, except in the early stages of plague, that is to say, before the disease has assumed an epidemic form, and while there is hope of the isolation of a small number of sick and contacts checking it from spreading.[35]

When the stringent measures – such as hospitalization, compulsory segregation, inspection of corpses, and use of police were withdrawn – people started cooperating with the administration. This resulted in the restoration of popular confidence, the enlistment of their co-operation to a greater extent, the diminution of attempts to conceal cases, the lessening of exodus on a considerable scale, and the lessening of the spread of infection. People also showed their co-operation by appointing their own men to inspect houses daily and reported the new arrivals to the local authorities.[36]

Discussion and conclusion

Like elsewhere in the country, administration's efforts towards oppressive plague-control measures clashed with the popular values and cultural beliefs of the people. Rumours were circulated saying that government had established camps where people were drugged, poisoned, and killed. As reported in the Indian Plague Commission Report of 1898–1899,[37] many believed that when a person went to the plague hospital, the person went there to die. It was the compulsions in anti-plague measures which constituted a barrier in winning the confidence of the people and getting their co-operation. The anti-plague measures of the government usually included mandatory hospitalization of victims, segregation of contacts, evacuation of epidemic localities, disinfection of plague affected houses, inspection of travellers, and detention of suspicious cases. However, the major opposition was towards hospitalization and segregation.

In Mysore in due course, compulsory segregation was abolished, subject to the condition that satisfactory arrangements were to be made for the disinfection of infected houses and for the separate treatment of patients. Additionally, satisfactory steps were to be taken to prevent the spread of plague to nearby localities.[38] Bangalore City had more compulsive measures, presumably because of the large number of plague deaths reported suddenly in the city. Compared to Bangalore, the Mysore Municipality seems to have organized the plague measures more 'wisely' – there was no compulsory removable to hospitals or segregation of contacts. Patients were encouraged to go to hospitals. But if they declined to go, they were treated in their own houses on condition that the infected house had to be disinfected on the death or recovery of the patient.[39]

The well-organized administrative machinery and existing public health facilities made it possible to tackle the plague epidemic in a more effective manner in Mysore Province. This is evident from the statistics that, from 1898 to 1918, each succeeding quinquennium recorded a steady decline in the plague mortality (see Table 1.3). The precautionary measures, as outlined by the Dewan and administration, provided a framework and guideline to the Municipalities of Bangalore and Mysore and to the Deputy Commissioners in charge of the districts. The gearing up of the entire administrative setup, when the disease struck in the neighbouring Dharwad district of Bombay Presidency, was remarkable. The leadership of Madhava Rao as Plague Commissioner and the police force under him added a new dimension and impetus to the governmental efforts to combat the epidemic. The health and town planning got a major boost, particularly in the cities of Bangalore and Mysore. Though strict measures evoked strong public resentments in the initial year of the outbreak, the administration was quick to understand the sentiments of public and change the plague policy. Considering the magnitude of the epidemic and the vast territory to be administered, the 'progressive state'[40] of Princely Mysore exhibited, rather effectively, both 'indigenous' and 'modern' ways of handling people's sensibilities and administrative firmness at the same time.

Table 1.3 Quinquennial averages of mortality from plague, 1898–1899 to 1922–1923, Mysore

Year	Average		Ratio per mille of population	Percentages of deaths to attacks
	Attacks	Deaths		
1898–1899 to 1902–1903	19490	14700	2.70	75.4
1903–1904 to 1907–1908	15902	11589	2.13	72.8
1908–1909 to 1912–1913	9669	6979	1.22	72.1
1913–1914 to 1917–1918	9555	6706	1.17	69.7
1917–1918 to 1922–1923	10157	1706	1.41	16.7

Source: *Mysore Gazetteer*: Compiled for Government, Volume IV. Administrative, (ed.) C. Hayavadana Rao, Government Press, Bangalore, 1929. p-445

Notes

1 'Indian Sanitary Proceedings', *India Office Library*, V7602, 1907, 1816–17.
2 L.F. Hirst, *The Conquest of Plague*, London: Oxford University Press, 1953, 300.
3 Ira Klein, 'Plague, Policy, and Popular Unrest in British India', *Modern Asian Studies*, 22(4), 1988, 723–55.
4 David Arnold, *Colonizing the Body: State Medicine and Epidemic Disease in Nineteenth-Century India*, Berkeley: University of California Press; New Delhi: Oxford University Press, 1993.
5 Total area of Mysore state was 27,936 square miles. It was divided into eight districts: Bangalore, Mysore, Kolar, Tumkur, Hassan, Kadur, Shimoga and Chitaldrug. Census of India, Vol. XXV, Mysore, Part 1, Report with Appendices, Bangalore: Government Central Printing Press, 1893.
6 C. Hayavadana Rao (ed.), *Mysore Gazetteer, Compiled for Government*, Vol. IV (Administrative), Bangalore: Government Press, 1929.
7 *Addresses of the Dewans of Mysore to the Dasara Representative Assembly, From 1881–1899*, Vol. I, Bangalore: Government Press, 1914, 255. (Karnataka State Archives).
8 In Dharwar, plague deaths till 1903–1904 amounted to 1,49,857, about 13 percent of the total population. *Gazetteer of Bombay Presidency*, Vol. XXII B, Dharwar and Savanur, Bombay: Government Press, 1905, 3.
9 V.P. Madhava Rao, *Report on Plague Operations in the Mysore State Excluding the Civil and Military Stations of Bangalore for the Year 1898–99* (from 1 July 1898 to 30 June 1899), Bangalore: Paragon Press, 1899, 13. (Karnataka State Archives).
10 *Report of the Administration of Mysore for the Four Years 1895–96 to 1898–99*, Bangalore: Mysore Government Central Press, 1900, 62. (Karnataka State Archives).
11 In Bombay City alone, the death toll from plague rose to 183,984 between 1896 to 1914. The oppressive measures of the administration met with strong protests from the public. For discussion, –see David Arnold, 'Touching the Body: Perspectives on the Indian Plague, 1896–1900', in Ranajit Guha (ed.), *Subaltern Studies*, Vol. V, New Delhi: Oxford University Press, 1988, 55–90 (reprinted in Ranajit Guha and Gayatri Spivak (eds.), *Selected Subaltern Studies*, New York: Oxford University Press, 1988, 391–426).

12 Madhava Rao carried on the plague-control measures with firmness and was considered an efficient administrator. He went on to become the Dewan of two provinces – first in Travancore (1904–1906) and later in Mysore (1906–1909).

13 'An Account of the Administration of the Mysore State During the year 1897–98', *Addresses of the Dewans of Mysore to the Dasara Representative Assembly, From 1881–1899*, Vol. I, Bangalore: Government Press, 1914, 239. Divisional Archives, Mysore (Karnataka State Archives).

14 Mysore was one of the largest princely states in India. For administrative purposes, Mysore State had been divided into eight districts, each presided over by a Deputy Commissioner. Every district consisted of several *Taluks* under the supervision of an *Amildar*. The *Amildar* was responsible for revenue administration, judicial work, and police work. The *Taluks* were sub-divided into *Hoblis*, which were under the supervision of *Sheikdars*, or Revenue Officers. For details, see James Manor, *Political Change in an Indian State: Mysore 1917–1955*. Australian National University Monograph on South Asia, No.2, Delhi: Manohar Publications, 1977.

15 *Report of the Administration of Mysore for the Four Years 1895–96 to 1898–99*, *Op.Cit.*, 63.

16 Annual Medical and Sanitary Report of Mysore, 1898–1899, General and Revenue Department, Government of HH the Maharaja of Mysore, 16 (Karnataka State Archives).

17 'The Report of the Indian Plague Commission', *British Medical Journal*, I(2157), 1902, 1093–8.

18 Annual Medical and Sanitary Report of Mysore, 1898–1899, General and Revenue Department, Government of HH the Maharaja of Mysore, 18 (Karnataka State Archives).

19 *Ibid.*

20 *Ibid.*, 65–6.

21 This measure was later abolished, following strong protests from the people, as discussed later in this chapter.

22 The administration of stimulants, both alcoholic and medicinal, were freely resorted to. Good nursing, combined with careful feeding and free stimulations, in the hope that the patient would survive the critical period, was found to be the most hopeful line of treatment.
    (*Report of the Administration of Mysore for the Four Years 1895–96 to 1898–99*, *Op. Cit.*, 66).

23 *Report of the Administration of Mysore for the Four Years 1895–96 to 1898–99*, *Op. Cit.*, xiv.

24 V.P. Madhava Rao, *Op.Cit.*, 21.

25 A case of plague was reported from the home of Hayagrivacharya. The patient was shifted to the hospital and the administration ordered disinfection of the house. Under the instruction of the British Inspector who visited the house, the disinfection procedure was carried out by the workers employed for the purpose, who belonged to lower castes. This hurt the religious sentiments of Hayagrivacharya. He felt that his house was defiled and committed suicide, blaming the oppressive plague measures. This incident was highlighted in the local newspapers and had repercussions in the Dharwar Municipality, resulting in the resignation of five elected members in protest.
    Reported in *Kesari*, 20 September 1898 (Maharashtra State Archives).

26 *Lok-Bandhu*, 11 September 1898; *Karnataka Vritta* (Dharwar), 20 September, 1898. (Maharashtra State Archives).

27 V.P. Madhava Rao, *Op.Cit*, 16.

28 *Ibid.*, 15.

29 *Ibid.*, 33.

30 Donald Rudolf Gustafson, *Mysore, 1881–1902, the Making of a Model State*, Unpublished Ph.D Thesis, Wisconsin, 1969, *as cited by* Leela B., 'Plague in Karnataka: 1896–1900', *Indica*, 36, 1999, The Heras Institute, Mumbai, 39–49.

31 The total number of vaccinations for the year 1897–1898 was 101,323. However, in the year of plague epidemic, it came down drastically to 36,515. "The very remarkable decline in the number of vaccinations in 1898–1899 was due to the prevalence of plague in some of the districts, while in others the people were under the impression that the vaccinators were inoculating for plague, and so decline to submit themselves to be vaccinated" – 'Mysore Administrative Report 1898–99', 161–2, (Karnataka State Archives).

32 Donald Rudolf Gustafson, *Mysore, 1881–1902, the Making of a Model State, Op. Cit.*, 294.

33 B. Lewis Rice, *Mysore: A Gazetteer Compiled for Government*, Vol. II, London: Archibald Constable & Company, Not Dated, 243.

34 Leela B., 'Plague in Karnataka: 1896–1900', *Indica*, 36, 1999 (The Heras Institute, Mumbai), 45.

35 *Report of the Administration of Mysore for the Four Years 1895–96 to 1898–99, Op. Cit.*, 65.

36 Reflections regarding this change in people's behaviour and involvement was noted in a diary of a District Plague Officer of Bangalore, and discussed in V.P. Madhava Rao, *Op.Cit.*, Extract from Diaries, vii.

37 'Indian Plague Commission 1898–99', in *Minutes of Evidences Taken by the Indian Plague Commission With Appendices*, Vol. I, Calcutta: Central Printing Office, 1900, 105.

38 *Report of the Administration of Mysore for the Four Years 1895–96 to 1898–99, Op. Cit.*, 65.

39 'The Report of the Indian Plague Commission', *Op.Cit.*, 1095.

40 Mysore was viewed as a 'progressive' Princely state because of its administrative modernization, state support for social services mainly for education and health, and the introduction of representative institutions such as Mysore Representative Assembly and later Legislative Council. For details, see Barbara Ramusack, *The Indian Princes and Their States: The New Cambridge History of India*, Cambridge: Cambridge University Press, 2004.

2 Addressing public health and sanitation in Mysore, 1881–1921

'Model' state and 'native' administrators

> By the substitution of Native for European subordinate medical staff, that department will be made more suitable for the requirements of the Native State.[1]
>
> Dewan of Mysore at the Mysore Representative Assembly (1884)

An important dimension of the history of public health administration in colonial India is the nature of interactions between the ideas of administration, the influence of Western medicine, and indigenous practices. It was a complex process, evolved over a period of time that reflected the concerns of the time and laid the seeds for 'modernizing' public health and sanitation measures in the country. The frequent outbreaks of epidemics and the loss of large number of lives became one of the drivers for introducing organized measures for disease control and environmental sanitation. However, the public health initiatives implemented during the colonial period have often been sceptically viewed as measures to protect British civilians and the army men. The colonial medical policy often focused attention to Europeans by neglecting the indigenous population.[2] This has credence in the fact that British lived in residentially segregated areas with good facilities for water supply and sanitation; the focus of medical services was on the detection and prevention of contagious diseases that could become a threat to the privileged.[3] At the same time, the main source of funding for hospitals and sanitary reforms were not from the Central Government, but were made by local authorities, charitable donations, and Municipalities. The Central Government mainly confined its role to legislations, leaving much of the responsibility for health and sanitary measures to the poorly funded and inexperienced local authorities.[4]

Nevertheless, the colonial authorities were instrumental for laying the seeds of a machinery that helped in developing an administrative structure for delivering public health services. This is more evident in the cities of the British Presidencies such as Bombay, Madras, and Calcutta. But, some of the Princely States,[5] such as Mysore and Travancore,[6] were able to incorporate appropriate measures for introducing modern sanitary practices and public health measures such as vaccination, while setting up administrative systems that were considered as 'models'. Particularly, in Mysore Princely State, this is interesting as it witnessed 50 years of direct British rule from 1831 to 1881, and then from 1881 onwards it was ruled by the local *Rajas*, the *Wodeyars*, after the British restored the throne to them by way of a subsidiary alliance. The developments in public health and sanitation in Mysore present a unique case for examining the blend in colonial and indigenous practices that shaped public health and sanitary administration in the province in the later part of the nineteenth century and early decades of the twentieth century.

Organization of public health administration

The reorganization of medical establishment came under serious consideration of the Mysore government since the rendition in 1881. This is reflected in the observation of the Dewan that the medical establishment "yet remain[ed] to be reformed".[7] Accordingly, the foundations of a system to provide medical services were laid in 1884:

> A complete and immediate reorganisation was contemplated, but in recognition of the inconvenience to all parties which would be caused by the reversion of number of medical subordinates to the Madras Government without previous notice, the Resident was of the opinion that the proposed reorganisation might be deferred for another year.[8]

In a letter dated 31 March 1881, the Resident communicated to the Madras government that on the expiry of the official year 1881–1882 "it would be necessary for the Madras Medical Subordinates employed in Mysore, except such as might elect for the local medical service, to revert to Madras."[9] Following this, the Madras administration promptly asked for a list of those medical subordinates who wished to opt for the local service of the Mysore government.

On its part, the Mysore government, after "careful consideration", was of the opinion that a medical service composed chiefly of duly qualified natives was best suited for the requirements of Mysore.[10] However, it was decided that the services of three Covenanted Medical Officers of the British service would be retained till 1886. After this period, it was considered that only two European Medical Officers would be sufficient in the State Service. One was to head the Medical Department and be the Chief Advisor to the Government, besides being in charge of all medical institutions in Bangalore. The second officer, a junior Medical Officer or a European carefully selected from the profession in England, was to be in charge of all medical institutions in Mysore, including discharging the functions as the '*Durbar* Surgeon'.[11]

The local Medical Officers were divided into three categories – Surgeons, Assistant Surgeons and Hospital Assistants. According to the appointment and promotion rules[12] for medical personnel, issued by R. Vijayindra Rao, Secretary to the Mysore government, Surgeons under the local medical service were to be always appointed by selection and if possible from the local Assistant Surgeons. The Surgeons were to be of three grades with specified salaries:

- 1st Grade – Rs. 500
- 2nd Grade – Rs. 450
- 3rd Grade – Rs. 350

To move from one grade to the next higher grade, one needed to complete five years of service. The Assistant Surgeons, who were under the administrative supervision of the Surgeons, were also placed under three grades:

- 1st Class Assistant Surgeon – Rs. 200
- 2nd Class Assistant Surgeon – Rs. 150
- 3rd Class Assistant Surgeon – Rs. 100

In 1887, a grade of Senior Hospital Assistants was created and in 1888 a grade of Sub-Assistant Surgeons of three classes on Rs. 80, 100 and 120 was introduced. The number of grades of Sub-Assistant Surgeons was subsequently reduced to two – 1st Class with a grade pay of Rs. 90 plus Rs. 30 as allowance, and 2nd Class with a grade pay of Rs. 70 plus Rs. 30 as allowance. For the special benefit of women doctors, a grade of *Apothecaries* was sanctioned, consisting of four classes on Rs. 75, 100, 125 and 150. Their promotion from one class to the next higher was regulated by approved service of five years. *Apothecaries* and Senior Hospital Assistants were declared eligible for promotion to the grades of Sub-Assistant Surgeons and Assistant Surgeons with grade pay ranging from Rs. 100 to 150.[13]

In order to attract best talents and qualified doctors, care was taken to ensure that the salary-scale for officers in the local medical service was similar to what was prevailing in the neighbouring Presidencies of Madras and Bombay. All persons entering the local medical service had to begin as 3rd Class Assistant Surgeons. However, there was exception for persons who had acquired professional experience elsewhere. Further, a basic qualification criterion was applied to all persons who were to be selected to the grade of Assistant Surgeons – they had to successfully complete the Madras M.B. Examination, or the L.M.S. Examination of Bombay or Madras.[14] The rules regarding service, gratuities, pensions, and leave, applicable to the offices of the local medical service, was the same as other offices of Mysore Public Service.

In 1881, Mysore State had only 24 hospitals and dispensaries, including two asylums – one for lunatics[15] and the other for people suffering from leprosy.[16] By 1918, the number of medical institutions increased up to 178 (see Table 2.1). It is important to mention here that the major attention of medical expansion was in the districts of Bangalore and Mysore. Out of 129 hospitals and dispensaries functioning in 1899, 47 were located in these two districts.[17] The Mysore government shouldered the major responsibility of funding the hospitals and dispensaries. Nearly 85 percent of the total cost for this was paid by the government, whereas the local sources (municipal, district, and local funds) contributed only 15 percent of the total cost of Rs. 3.86, 752 in the year 1897–1898.[18]

Another area of focus was the starting of special dispensaries for women and children and appointment of midwives. At the time of rendition, there were no qualified midwives in the state. A few selected women were sent to Madras for training, with scholarship, and by 1891, the Department had 19 trained midwives.[19] In his address to the Mysore Representative Assembly in 1895, Dewan K.Seshadri Iyer, stated:

Table 2.1 Growth of medical institutions in Mysore, 1881–1923

Medical institutions	1881	1891	1901	1911	1918	1923
State public-general and special hospitals and dispensaries	8	9	15	15	26	28
State non-public,such as jail, military and Public Work Department	–	6	6	8	8	9
Local funds and municipal dispensaries	16	81	113	116	128	146
Private aided				3	4	7
Private non-aided				2	2	3
Railway dispensaries				5	10	7
Total	24	96	134	149	178	200

Source: *Mysore Gazetteers*, compiled for Government, Vol.4 (Administrative), Edited by C. Hayavadana Rao, Bangalore, 1927–1930. p-432

His Highness fully appreciating the importance of Lady Dufferin's philanthropic movement directed the training and employment of midwives all over the country and the opening of special dispensaries for women and children. All but three taluks out of 66 have been provided with midwives and 5 dispensaries for women and children have been opened in district head-quarter towns.[20]

A medical school was established in 1881 for training the Hospital Assistants, but this was closed in 1886. The practice was to give scholarships to students to go through a course, either in Madras or Bombay Medical Colleges. Due to constraints, such as providing accommodation to students, Madras Presidency expressed inability to admit Mysore students. Following this, the Government of Mysore sanctioned a scheme, in April 1917, at Bangalore to train Sub-Assistant Surgeons required for service in the state, and the Mysore Medical School started functioning from 1 July 1917. Though this medical school was located at Bangalore, it was named as Mysore Medical School.[21] At the time of its inception, it had 16 students, with the Medical Officer In-Charge of Victoria Hospital[22] acting as its Principal.[23]

The government, in July 1918, again sanctioned the reorganization of the department at an additional recurring cost of Rs. 80,000 per annum by adding to the number of superior officers and also revising the pay of the several grades.[24] Excluding the Senior Surgeon, the number of Surgeons was increased to 16 and they were appointed under six pay grades (see Table 2.2).

The strength of Assistant Surgeons was increased from 29 to 34 permanent, and one temporary, and they were placed in two grades of pay – 1st Class with a grade pay of Rs 200–20–360 and 2nd Class with a grade pay of Rs 120–10–200. The

Table 2.2 Pay scales of surgeons, 1918

Grade	Number	Pay
1st Class	1	Rs. 800–50–900
2nd Class	2	Rs. 700–50–800
3rd Class	3	Rs. 500–25–700
4th Class	3	Rs. 500
5th Class	3	Rs. 450
6th Class	4	Rs. 400

Source: *Mysore Gazetteers*, compiled for Government, Vol.4 (Administrative), Edited by C. Hayavadana Rao, Bangalore, 1927–1930. p-424

grade of Assistant Surgeons was abolished. The pay of the Lady Apothecaries was raised from Rs. 75-25-5-150 to Rs. 75–5–200.

It is interesting to note that there were 50 medical officers constituting the gazetted ranks in July 1935 under the Mysore government. Of them, ten had obtained professional qualifications in British universities, and two had undertaken foreign travel to study the working of medical institutions in the different countries they visited. The rest were graduates in medicine and surgery from Indian universities.[25] To improve the efficiency of the department, the government encouraged officers and young men of promise by offering scholarships to study in foreign universities to obtain higher qualification, and to specialize in their profession.[26]

In 1919, the Government of Mysore appointed a committee with the Senior Surgeon as President, consisting of three official and three non-official members, to reorganize the Medical Department for improving its functioning. The Committee made many recommendations,[27] some of which were:

(a) Opening of 102 new dispensaries within the next five years to be manned by Sub-Assistant Surgeons.
(b) Development of District Hospitals.
(c) Construction of new building for the Lunatic Asylum.
(d) Extension of medical relief through *Unani* and *Ayurvedic* dispensaries.[28]
(e) Opening of Maternity Centres in every district headquarter, with facility for training *Dayis* in midwifery.
(f) Establishing a Medical College at an initial and recurring cost of Rs 8,25, 000 and Rs 60,100, respectively.
(g) Fixing a program of expenditure for the next five years, along the following lines – first year: Rs. 9,27,012; second year: Rs. 9,55,024; third year: Rs. 10,13,036; fourth year: Rs. 10,71,048; and fifth year: Rs. 11,34,064.

The government approved most of these recommendations. The action taken report shows that 34 dispensaries had opened during the five years from 1920 to 1925; a combined *Ayurvedic* and *Unani* dispensary was established at Shimoga; and scholarships were provided to students to pursue *Unani* system of medicine in Tibbi College, Delhi (a college setup for imparting education and training in *Unani* medicine).[29]

Organization of Sanitary Department

Two statements from the Dewan of Mysore amply illustrate the concerns of the administration on the sanitary front. In 1893, the Dewan said in the Representative Assembly:

> The want had long been felt of a separate qualified Engineer who could give his exclusive attention to developing effective measures for the sanitation of the Cities of Mysore and Bangalore and of the more populous towns in the State as well as to designing and carrying out works of water-supply and drainage wherever required.[30]

For this purpose, Standish Lee was appointed, under the designation of 'Sanitary Engineer', in 1893. Dewan Seshadri Iyer further emphasized the government's commitment towards improving sanitation in 1895, by stating:

> Special attention to sanitation was an important feature of His Highness' reign. In addition to sanitary works carried out by the various District Fund Boards and Municipalities, His Highness devoted the large sum of Rs. 27, 15, 221 from State Revenues for the improved sanitation of the capital cities of Mysore and Bangalore and of the larger moffusil towns throughout the State.[31]

Thus, government made considerable efforts to organize the sanitary administration in the State. For the efficient sanitary administration, a Department of Public Health was constituted in 1907, with the Senior Surgeon as Ex-Officio Sanitary Commissioner, and a full-time Deputy Sanitary Commissioner to assist in administering the department.[32] The state was divided into three divisions for the purpose of sanitary administration, that is, Western, Eastern, and Southern Divisions. Each Division was under a Divisional Sanitary Officer. At the district level, District Sanitary Officers were appointed, and Sanitary Inspectors and Assistant Sanitary Inspectors were made in charge of each Taluk and Municipality. In 1909–1910, the post of Divisional Sanitary Officers were abolished and the pay scales of the District Sanitary Officers was raised to attract qualified persons. Realizing that the sanitary reforms in the State had not progressed, through further reorganization, in 1917 a full-time Sanitary Commissioner was appointed as the head of the department. In 1919, the number of positions for senior officials and their pay scales were revised. However, many positions could not be filled due to non-availability of enough qualified persons. The lack of funds at the Taluk and Municipal levels also delayed appointments.[33]

Another important introduction in sanitary reforms in Mysore was the setting up of the Advisory Sanitary Boards in 1907 – Central Sanitary Board for the state and a District Sanitary Board for each district. The Central Sanitary Board consisted of the Sanitary Commissioner, the Revenue Commissioner, the Chief Engineer, the Deputy Sanitary Commissioner, and the Sanitary Engineer. Amongst its responsibilities, the Central Sanitary Board examined the schemes submitted by the District Sanitary Boards and advised the government on their desirability. Likewise, the District Sanitary Board consisted of the Deputy Commissioner, Divisional Sanitary Officer, District Engineer, District Medical Officer, District Sanitary Officer and two members of the Municipal or Local Fund Board. The District Sanitary Board were expected to advise Municipalities and district administration with regard to schemes for improving sanitary conditions. Schemes with a budget of less than Rs. 1000 were placed under purview of the District Sanitary Board, while schemes which required higher budgets were sent to the consideration and approval of the Central Sanitary Board. However, there were limitations in the role and utility of the sanitary boards, as they had only an advisory role. This concern was expressed by the Sanitary Commissioner, T.V. Arumugum Mudaliar, in his Annual Sanitary Report of 1913, wherein he stated:

> The Board [Central] is at present merely an advisory body and can only examine such schemes as are referred to it for opinion. With a view to providing for initiative by the Board certain rules have been proposed and when these are approved by the Government the Board will be in a position to *investigate* and *suggest* sanitary schemes and measures.[34]

It was also decided to have a Public Health Institute and Laboratory attached to the Department.[35] In 1912, a training course for Sanitary Inspectors, with a duration of six months, was started at the Public Health Institute, Bangalore. This course was modelled as that of the Sanitary Inspectors of Madras.

The Sanitary Department had the major responsibility to scrutinize and compile birth and death returns, supervise vaccination, and control epidemics. As part of its duties, the Sanitary Department also made efforts to prevent the cremation or burial of dead bodies by the side of streams, *nallas*, etc. The senior officials had to carry out regular inspections of the sanitary works.

Subsequently, the nature and scope of the duties increased considerably and the control of plague operations for which there was a Special Plague Commissioner from 1898 to 1902 was made part of the Sanitary Commissioner's duties in 1902.[36] Other sanitary works pertained to relieving congested areas, opening out conservancy lanes and roads, constructing and repairing drains and tunnels, repairing and sinking fresh water wells, filling-up trenches and pits, removing rank vegetation, etc., and these were undertaken mostly by the Municipalities.[37]

An important development in the Sanitary Administration was the opening of the Epidemic Diseases Hospital in Bangalore in 1891.[38] Originally known as *Chattram* Hospital, and later named as 'Hospital for Infectious Diseases', it was located adjacent to the Railway Station. It was essentially meant for accommodating and treating of cases of infectious or communicable diseases amongst the locals and also those who arrived in the city by train. In 1897, the Epidemic Diseases Regulation was passed in Mysore.[39] Another landmark measure in sanitary administration was the passing of the Mysore Village Sanitary Regulation in 1898,[40] which provided powers to the government to make rules to regulate the conservancy of villages, for protection and periodical examination of wells and water supply, and to punish those who violated the rules defining the sanitary measures. Further, the constitution of the Village Improvement Committees encouraged voluntary involvement and labour contributions from villagers to maintain cleanliness and hygiene in the village precincts. Likewise, City Improvement Committees were also set up in Bangalore and Mysore to inspect localities that had congested housing. Under Land Acquisition Regulation,[41] steps were taken by the city administration to acquire the properties required for opening out conservancy lines and abate overcrowding.[42] With a view to ensure adequate sanitation during *jatras*, cattle fairs and exhibitions, the government passed an order on 7 June 1913 which stated that

> when applying for permission to hold special *jatras*, Deputy Commissioners should invariably submit for the information of Government a brief report as to the sanitary arrangements proposed to be made for the occasion.[43]

However, the sanitation measures focused mostly on urban areas, neglecting the villages. The Sanitary Commissioner, in his report in 1913, admitted that

> Through lack of funds and proper organizations for dealing with village sanitation there has been no progress in village improvements worth recording. . . . The constitution of village agencies recently ordered by Government will, I believe, tend, among other things, to place this question of Village Sanitation on a more satisfactory basis.[44]

He went on to emphasize the importance of initiating an organized attempt to improve and protect rural water supply to safeguard against outbreaks of epidemics. The importance given to rural sanitation is evident from the address of Mirza M. Ismail, who was the Dewan of Mysore between 1926 and 1941, to the Mysore Representative Assembly in 1928.[45] He observed that the Government of Mysore cannot rest satisfied until those living in rural areas, who formed the bulk of the population, had clean drinking water and a dispensary with sufficient stock of medicines.

Epidemic administration: vaccination

The Sanitary Report of the Deputy Commissioner of Chitaldrug district in 1890, based on his experience in Talagatta Village in the Holalkere Taluk, highlights the opposition from villages to the vaccination programme of the Mysore government:

> Accompanied by the Deputy Inspector of Vaccination and the Taluk vaccinator and also the *Amildar*, I went to that village to see as many of the unprotected children as possible vaccinated before my own eyes. No sooner did we go into the village and the villagers came to know the object with which we had come

than they shut their doors against us. No amount of good advice and moral persuasion would induce them to open their doors and bring out their children for our inspection, and it was only after some 3 or 4 children brought by the *Patel* had been somewhat forcibly vaccinated in my presence, that the villagers were induced to think that there was no use of their opposing us any further, and about 20 children were then voluntarily brought out and vaccinated in about an hour's time. Finding therefore that people, who could offer so much opposition in spite of the presence of the *Amildar* and myself on the spot, could do it a hundred-fold when the vaccinator, a poor, ill-paid official, went about in the Taluk, alone and unaccompanied even by a peon, I issued a circular to all *Amildars* in the district to give the vaccinator all needful assistance in his work.[46]

During the period 1895 to 1900, Mysore state recorded considerable mortality from diseases such as plague, smallpox, cholera, etc. (see Table 2.3). Referring to this scenario, Brigade-Surgeon Lt. Colonel P.H. Benson, Senior Surgeon and Sanitary Commissioner of Mysore Government, in his Annual Medical and Sanitary Report of 1895–1896, while quoting his predecessor, reiterated:

I firmly believe that the only measures that will make any serious diminution or anything approaching a satisfactory one in the death rate from this disease [smallpox] is a Compulsory Vaccination Act combined with measures to provide an abundant and unobjectionable supply of lymph.[47]

Benson again expressed his frustration the following year:

It is very regrettable in the nineteenth century and in a civilized country to have to record such a death rate from a disease which is perhaps of all diseases the most preventable as is evidenced by the small mortality that occurs from this disease in Germany, where, with a population of 27,000,000 there were only 50 deaths; such a result, however, cannot be expected until vaccination and re-vaccination are made compulsory.[48]

Table 2.3 Mortality and causes of death in Mysore, 1895–1900

Year	Death rate per mille of population						
	Cholera	Smallpox	Fevers	Bowel complaints	Injuries	All other causes	Total
1895–1896	0.11	0.59	7.50	0.99	0.24	3.86	13.28
1896–1897	0.96	1.38	7.55	1.01	0.23	3.88	15.01
1897–1898	0.49	1.49	12.16	1.50	0.25	4.35	20.24
1898–1899	0.11	0.88	8.63	1.59	0.92	6.96	19.00
1899–1900	0.03	0.72	7.55	1.25	0.25	6.85	16.64

Source: Annual Medical and Sanitary Report of Mysore for the Year 1899–1900, General and Revenue Departments (Karnataka State Archives), p-3

P.H. Benson's frustration was justified by the increasing mortality from smallpox. In the year 1895–1896, the number of deaths from smallpox was 2853, and this went up to 6676 deaths in 1896–1897. The ratio of death per mille of population was 1.38 (the highest was in Chitaldrug District – 2.29).[49] The following year also witnessed a high mortality from smallpox with 7203 deaths. Benson was desperately seeking for a Compulsory Vaccination Act. Once this was done, he was confident that the epidemic could be combated. He was convinced that Mysore had the facility required for supporting compulsory vaccination and just an Act was needed to ensure regular inoculation:

> We have at present in the Vaccine Institute[50] which is capable of supplying any amount of lano-line paste manufactured direct from calf lymph according to Surgeon Major King's method, so that the Compulsory Vaccination Act is all we want.[51]

From the concerns raised and the pleas for Compulsory Vaccination Act expressed by P.H. Benson, it is evident that the thrust for epidemic control came from the British Officers stationed in the state. In 1880, an Act was passed for the compulsory vaccination of children in Municipalities and Cantonments. Subsequently, a Regulation passed in 1906 made vaccination compulsory in the state that gave powers to the government to declare compulsory vaccination in any local area in the state.[52]

In 1881, at the time of rendition, the Vaccination Department was working under the Department of Public Health, and under the supervision of the Senior Surgeon. There were three types of vaccinators – 1st Class Vaccinators with a monthly pay of Rs. 15; 2nd Class Vaccinators with a monthly pay of Rs. 12; and 3rd Class Vaccinators with a monthly pay of Rs. 10. Each Vaccinator was expected to vaccinate ten persons for each rupee of their pay or suffer a proportional fine.[53] However, the conditions imposed by the government on Vaccinators led to fudging of vaccination statistics in connivance with village officials. Taking this into consideration, the stipulation regarding the number of monthly vaccinations to be carried out by each Vaccinator was later withdrawn.[54]

There were 84 Taluk level Vaccinators in 1880–1881, and this figure went up to 161 Vaccinators and 8 Deputy Inspectors by 1923–1924. There was a reserve Vaccinator for each district for undertaking emergency work, whenever necessary. The entire cost of vaccination was met by the Mysore government, except in Municipalities of Bangalore and Mysore, which had their own Vaccinators. A cash award was instituted to the most active Vaccinator in each district. In a major revamp of the Vaccination Department in 1907, a decision was taken that "the staff vaccinators were to be replaced by a better class of specially trained men".[55] As men with requisite training were not available, arrangements were made to select suitable men and have them trained.

To administer the vaccine programme effectively, a preliminary survey of 'unprotected' children was undertaken. In Bangalore, Mysore, and Kolar Gold Fields, census was taken in the year 1914–1915. The village functionaries (*Patels*) were informed about arrival of the Vaccinator in their village well in advance, and it was their responsibility to have all 'unprotected' children ready for vaccination on the specified date. After the vaccination in the village, the *Patel* had to send a report to the Deputy Inspector of Vaccination and also to the *Amildar* (Taluk level official). The Vaccinator was required to submit a task-completed report at the end of each month to the Deputy Inspector of Vaccination.[56] District Sanitary Officers, District Sanitary Assistants, and Deputy Inspectors had to routinely visit the field to examine if the persons who were vaccinated bore the marks of successful vaccination.

Administering an epidemic: the case of influenza pandemic of 1918

The Sanitary Commissioner of India, F. Norman White, in his preliminary report on influenza, observed:

> Influenza within the space of four or five months was responsible for the death of 2 percent of the total population of British India, the percentage of persons falling victim varying between 5.7 in the Central Provinces and 0.4 in Bengal. As regards the incidence of the disease in Native States but little information is, at present, available, with the single exception of Mysore. The total number of deaths ascribed to influenza in Mysore, in 1918, was 1,27,651, which is equivalent to a death rate of 22.37 per thousand.[57]

The fact that only Mysore could provide timely information on influenza mortality gives credence to the administrative efficiency of the state even during a major public health crisis. The administration acted swiftly and firmly in tackling the pandemic through a set of measures that addressed the health concerns, along with financial support. Daily messages and weekly reports were sought in order to monitor the situation and have action plans. The memorandum issued by the government specified the responsibilities of the Senior Surgeon and Sanitary Commissioner, along with the Deputy Commissioners of Districts and Presidents of Municipalities. The instructions issued by the Chief Secretary and the specific guidelines from the Senior Surgeon and the Sanitary Commissioner provided a framework for the relief measures. The stern action enforced by the administration to regulate the prices of essential food grains during the influenza pandemic also formed part of the administrative initiatives to tackle the influenza pandemic. While addressing the Representative Assembly on 17 October 1918, the then-Dewan M. Visvesvaraya warned the merchants responsible for the sudden shortage of food grains that had created a famine-like situation:

> The strong hand of Government must always be in evidence and continue to interfere whenever any section of the community tries to take advantage of the difficulties of the public.[58]

The Proceedings of the Representative Assembly thus indicate the free and frank discussions on the effectiveness of relief measures and the government's willingness to listen to the complaints and act accordingly. Considering the magnitude of the epidemic and the vast area and population under its jurisdiction, the Mysore government and its well-organized administrative machinery provides insights into how it was able to tackle the challenges of the pandemic.[59]

Concluding observations

While appreciating and adopting the modern medical practices, the Princely state was determined to appoint qualified 'native' people in the medical and sanitary departments, instead of European subordinate medical staff and even those deputed from the neighbouring Madras Presidency. This was one policy followed with 'careful consideration' by Mysore administration after the rendition. Considerable investments were made in modernizing the medical and sanitary services in the last decades of the nineteenth century and early part of the twentieth century. At the same time, the administrative setup and procedures introduced during the 50 years of direct colonial rule (1831–1881) established a machinery which was 'modern' in outlook and could adapt to the challenges. This was evident in the manner in which Mysore addressed the plague epidemic and influenza pandemic. One of the critical features of the Mysore administration was the enhancement of the capability of 'native' medical personnel by having them trained abroad. Many of the legislations, which were introduced by the British to combat epidemics, were timely incorporated in the state, which also helped in streamlining and strengthening the epidemic administration. Another important feature that reflects the uniqueness of Mysore was the willingness of the government to allow free expression of people's concerns through the Representative Assembly (later, the Legislative Council). Immediately after assuming power by the *Wodeyars*, the Dewan of Mysore said:

> His Highness' Government will be glad to receive any observations and suggestions which you may wish to make in the public interests, and I need not assure you that they will meet with every consideration.[60]

This statement of its Dewan clearly posits, not only the importance attached by the State for public participation in the political process, but also its willingness to listen to the public voices, adding to its credence to be considered as a 'model' state. This approach, in turn, encouraged the adoption of innovative measures and application of modern science in developing medical institutions, health and sanitary infrastructure, and legislations for laying the foundations of a 'progressive' public health and sanitary administration in one of the largest Princely states of British India.

Notes

1 Statement of K. Seshadri Iyer, Dewan of Mysore, in the *Dasara* Session of the Mysore Representative Assembly on 1 October 1884, *Proceedings of the Mysore Representative Assembly, Addresses of the Dewans of Mysore to the Dasara Representative Assembly, From 1881–1899*, Vol. I, Bangalore: Government Press, 1914 (Karnataka State Archives), 38.

2 David Arnold, 'Medical Priorities and Practice in Nineteenth Century British India', *South Asia Research*, 5, 1985, 167–83; Radhika Ramasubban, *Public Health and Medical Research in India: Their Origins and Development Under the Impact of British Colonial Policy*, Stockholm: SAREC, 1982.

3 Mark Harrison, *Public Health in British India: Anglo-Indian Preventive Medicine 1859–1914*, Cambridge: Cambridge University Press, 1994; Sumit Guha, 'Nutrition, Sanitation, Hygiene, and the Likelihood of Death: The British Army in India c 1870–1920', *Population Studies*, 47(3), 1993, 385–401; Monica Dasgupta, 'Public Health in India: An Overview', *World Bank Policy Research Working Paper*, Number 3787, Washington, DC: World Bank, 2005.

4 David Arnold, 'Medical Priorities and Practice in Nineteenth Century British India', 1985, *Op.Cit.*; Biswamoy Pati and Mark Harrison,'Health, Medicine and Empire: Perspectives on Colonial India' (Introduction), in Biswamoy Pati and Mark Harrison (eds.), *Health, Medicine and Empire: Perspectives on Colonial India*, Hyderabad: Orient Longman, 2001, 1–36.

5 Princely or native states were those areas of India that were under the administration of Indian kings and not under the British Crown. However, the defence and foreign policies of these native states were controlled by the colonial government. But, at the same time, these native states had considerable autonomy in internal administration. In 1910, there were about 680 native states, and constituted about 45 percent of the total area of British India (excluding Burma and Sind), and 23 percent of its population in 1911.

6 Some native states were greatly committed to investments in education and healthcare during the colonial period. Mysore introduced the smallpox vaccination in 1806, while Travancore had a policy of free primary education in 1817. In an analysis of direct and indirect colonial rule in India, it is observed that the quality of governance in the colonial period had a significant and persistent effect on post-colonial outcomes. The provinces that were under direct rule had lower levels of access to schools, health centres, and roads in the post-colonial period – for details, see Lakshmi Iyer, 'Direct Versus Indirect Colonial Rule in India: Long-term Consequences', *The Review of Economics and Statistics*, XCII(4), 2010, 693–713.

7 Address of the Dewan to the Mysore Representative Assembly on 7 October 1881, a few months after the *Wodeyars* assumed power in the province. *Proceedings of the Mysore Representative Assembly, Addresses of the Dewans of Mysore to the Dasara Representative Assembly, From 1881–1899*, Vol. I, Bangalore: Government Press, 1914 (Karnataka State Archives), 6.

8 *Proceedings of the Dewan to His Highness the Maharaja of Mysore* (General), dated 5 May 1884, 1 (Karnataka State Archives).

9 *Ibid.*, 1.

10 *Ibid.*, 1.

11 *Ibid.*, 1.

12 *Ibid.*, 1–2.

13 C. Hayavadana Rao (ed.), *Mysore Gazetteer, Compiled for the Government*, Vol. IV (Administrative), Bangalore: Government Press, 1929, 423.

14 *Proceedings of the Dewan to His Highness the Maharaja of Mysore* (General), *Op.Cit.*, 2. *Note*: The higher teaching of medicine in colonial India was concentrated at Calcutta, Bombay, Madras, and Lahore. The Bombay and Madras Universities granted a degree of Licentiate in Medicine and Surgery (LMS) and a degree of Medical Bachelor (MB). The most striking difference in the LMS offered was that the general educational qualification was lower at Bombay than elsewhere and the course was shorter at Madras than elsewhere. At Madras, the preliminary qualification was the same in each case, but the course for a Bachelor's degree was longer – R. Nathan CIE, Office of the Director-General of Education in India. *Progress of Education in India: 1897–98 to 1901–02*, Fourth Quinquennial Review, Vol. 1, Calcutta: Office of the Superintendent of Government Printing, 1904, 235.

15 Lunatic Asylum, started in a hospital in Bangalore in 1847, expanded over the years and came to be regarded as unique amongst the mental hospitals in British India by practicing "modern methods of diagnosis and treatment". The Mysore Lunacy Regulation was passed in 1916. Mysore was the only Princely state to have an asylum for those considered as insane. For details, see Sanjeev Jain, 'Psychiatry and Confinement in India', in Roy Porter and David Wright (eds.), *The Confinement of the Insane: International Perspectives, 1800–1965*, Cambridge: Cambridge University Press, 2003, 273–98.

16 An asylum for those suffering from leprosy of the Cantonment and Pettah of Bangalore was built under the directions of Mark Cubbon in the year 1845. In 1857 the facility was expanded – 'Copy of Replies by J. Kirkpatrick, Surgeon to the Mysore Commission (dated Bangalore, March 1864), 485, in *Medical Reports Upon the Character and Progress of Leprosy in the East Indies: Being Answers to Interrogatories Drawn Up by the Royal College of Physicians, London*, Calcutta: J.L. Kingham Foreign Department Press, 1865.

17 *Mysore Administrative Report*, 1898–99 (Karnataka State Archives), 154.

18 *Ibid.*, 156.

19 *Mysore Gazetteer, Compiled for the Government*, Vol. IV (Administrative), *Op.Cit.*, 433.

20 Statement of K. Seshadri Iyer, Dewan of Mysore, in the Dasara Session of the Mysore Representative Assembly on 1 October 1895, in *Proceedings of the Mysore Representative Assembly, Addresses of the Dewans of Mysore to the Dasara Representative Assembly, From 1881–1899*, Vol. I, Bangalore: Government Press, 1914 (Karnataka State Archives), 206.

   For a detailed discussion on women's hospitals and midwives, refer: Barbara Ramusack, 'Women's Hospitals and Midwives in Mysore, 1870–1920: Princely or Colonial Medicine', in Waltraud Ernst and Biswamoy Pati (eds.), *India's Princely States: People, Princes and Colonialism*, London: Routledge, 2007, 173–93.

21 Initially, the students of Mysore Medical School were provided teaching facilities at Victoria Hospital in Bangalore and the course was four years for them to be qualified to become Licentiate in Medical Practise (LMP). Subsequently, in 1924–1925, the Mysore Medical School was made a college, called Mysore Medical College, and was affiliated to University of Mysore.

22 Victoria Hospital was built at a cost of Rs. 7,50,000, and was opened on 8 December 1890 by Lord Curzon, the then-viceroy and governor general of India. It had an administrative block with eight pavilions to accommodate a hundred in-patients to begin with, an operation theatre, and a laboratory –For details, refer: *Mysore Gazetteer, Compiled for the Government*, Vol. IV (Administrative), *Op.Cit.*

23 *Mysore Gazetteer, Compiled for the Government*, Vol. IV (Administrative), *Op.Cit.*, 425.

24 *Ibid.*, 423–4.

25 *Ibid.*, 425.

26 *Ibid.*, 426.

27 *Ibid.*, 437.

28 The Indigenous Hospital in Mysore City, started in 1892, had both *Ayurvedic* and *Unani* branches. Later an *Ayurvedic* College was started in 1908.

   For a critical appraisal of growth and expansion of *Ayurveda* and *Unani* medicine in Mysore State, refer: Guy Attewell, 'Compromised: Making Institutions and Indigenous Medicine in Mysore State, Circa 1908–1940', *Cult Med Psychiatry*, 38, 2014, 369–86.

29 *Mysore Gazetteer, Compiled for the Government*, Vol. IV (Administrative), *Op.Cit.*, 438.

30 Statement of K. Seshadri Iyer, Dewan of Mysore, in the *Dasara* Session of the Mysore Representative Assembly on 23 October 1893, in *Proceedings of the Mysore Representative Assembly, Addresses of the Dewans of Mysore to the Dasara Representative Assembly, From 1881–1899*, Vol. I, Bangalore: Government Press, 1914 (Karnataka State Archives), 164.

31 *Ibid.*, 206.

32 Mysore Administration Report, 1907, 61 (Karnataka State Archives).

33 *Ibid.*, 62.
34 Annual Sanitary Report for the Year 1913, General and Revenue Departments, Mysore, 7 (Karnataka State Archives).
35 Early in 1899, the Bacteriological Laboratory was opened and, according to the *Mysore Administrative Report of 1898–99* (page 161), it was the "finest and most completely equipped laboratory in India" at that time. Public Health Institute, Bangalore, was founded in 1911. Its major responsibilities were to provide laboratory support for investigations on outbreak of epidemics. With the establishment of the Public Health Institute, the Bacteriological Laboratory was merged into it –*Mysore Gazetteer, Compiled for the Government*, Vol. IV (Administrative), *Op.Cit.*, 453.
36 *Mysore Gazetteer, Compiled for the Government*, Vol. IV (Administrative), *Op.Cit.*, 427.
37 Mysore Administration Report, 1903, 70 (Karnataka State Archives).
38 *Mysore Gazetteer, Compiled for the Government*, Vol. IV (Administrative), *Op.Cit.*, 442.
39 *Proceedings of the Mysore Representative Assembly* (Karnataka State Archives), 8 October 1897, *Addresses of the Dewans of Mysore to the Dasara Representative Assembly, From 1881–1899*, Vol. I, Bangalore: Government Press, 1914, 235.
40 *Mysore Gazetteer, Compiled for the Government*, Vol. IV (Administrative), *Op.Cit.*, 450.
41 In 1857, the British enacted a land acquisition legislation that applied to the Presidencies and the whole of British India. Act VI of 1857 repealed all previous enactments relating to land acquisition, and its objective was to make better provision for the acquisition of land needed for public purposes within the territories in the possession and under the governance of the East India Company. Subsequently, it was amended in 1861 and then again in 1863 and in 1870. The enactment of the 1870 law, for the first time brought a mechanism for settlement (the reference to a civil court for compensation). This was eventually replaced by the Land Acquisition Act of 1894. However, the 1894 law did not apply to the Princely states of Hyderabad, Mysore, and Travancore, which enacted their own land acquisition legislations.
42 Annual Sanitary Report for the Year 1913, *Op.Cit.*, 7.
43 *Ibid.*
44 *Ibid.*
45 *Addresses of the Dewans of Mysore to the Mysore Representative Assembly, From 1913 to 1938, 4 Volumes*, Mysore: Government Branch Press (Karnataka State Archives).
46 *Annual Medical and Sanitary Report of Mysore for the Year 1890*, General and Revenue Department, Government of HH the Maharaja of Mysore, 12 (Karnataka State Archives).
47 *Annual Medical and Sanitary Report of Mysore for the Year 1895–96*, General and Revenue Department, Government of HH the Maharaja of Mysore, 3 (Karnataka State Archives).
48 *Annual Medical and Sanitary Report of Mysore for the Year 1896–97*, General and Revenue Department, Government of HH the Maharaja of Mysore, 8 (Karnataka State Archives).
49 *Ibid.*, 9.
50 The Vaccine Institute was established at Bangalore in 1892, initially as a temporary measure and later made permanent in 1896 (Mysore Administration Report, 1892, 162 (Karnataka State Archives).
51 *Annual Medical and Sanitary Report of Mysore for the Year 1895–96*, *Op.Cit.*, 9.
52 *Mysore Gazetteer, Compiled for the Government*, Vol. IV (Administrative), *Op.Cit.*, 456.
53 *Ibid.*, 453.
54 *Ibid.*, 454.
55 Mysore Administration Report, 1907, 62 (Karnataka State Archives).
56 Mysore Administration Report, 1914 (Karnataka State Archives).
57 *A Preliminary Report on the Influenza Epidemic of 1918 in India*, Simla: Government Monotype Press, 1919, 5 (Wellcome Library, London).

58 *Proceedings of Mysore Representative Assembly, Dasara Session, October 1918*, Bangalore: Government Press, 1919, 3.
59 T.V. Sekher, 'Public Health Administration in Princely Mysore: Tackling the Influenza Pandemic of 1918', in Waltraud Ernst and Biswamoy Pati (eds.), *India's Princely States: People, Princes and Colonialism*, London: Routledge, 2007, 194–211.
60 Statement of C.V. Rungacharlu, Dewan of Mysore, in the *Dasara* Session of the Mysore Representative Assembly on 7 October 1881, in *Proceedings of the Mysore Representative Assembly, Addresses of the Dewans of Mysore to the Dasara Representative Assembly, From 1881–1899*, Vol. I, Bangalore: Government Press, 1914 (Karnataka State Archives), 1.

Section 2

The Orissan states

Biswamoy Pati

3 Princely maladies

Leprosy

'World's first leprosy vaccine, from Indian lab, to go on trial'[1]
Times of India, 21 August 2016

It is indeed difficult to comprehend why the stigma and discrimination against 'leprosy' has had such a long life. The 'Otherization', 'seclusion', 'confinement', the campaigns and efforts to 'purge' from society those affected with leprosy is rather well known. As a disease, leprosy has been located diversely in different belief systems. Thus, the world of the Adivasis in colonial India, as we are told, explains it as the handiwork of the evil spirits. In fact, this stereotype constructed by the colonial 'civilizing mission' has been sustained in post-colonial India. However, the efforts to treat it as a disease amongst some Adivasis clearly illustrate complexities that are often ignored. Brahminical Hinduism normally explained leprosy as 'God's curse' – while the Ayurvedic system located it as a disease and the reference to the use of Chaulmogra oil being used to comfort those affected by the disease perhaps illustrates its location as a disease.

We are told about late medieval Europe, where Jews were located as its major carriers. Additionally, Christian missionaries in colonial India sometimes explained it as a disease of the 'soul', although Jesus 'curing' those who had leprosy is well known. As for Islam, it considers leprosy as a disease of the 'body'. Though the system of locating the cause of leprosy seems to be explained in diverse ways, this effort to interpret and explain it in binarized terms is difficult to sustain. After all, the body/soul dichotomy – viz. Christianity/Islam – seems to be too farfetched. Going beyond what has been mentioned, leprosy's visibility, which indicated that something was wrong with those having it, is as old as its existence.

Two basic aspects become relevant to the social historian of health and medicine when it comes to studying the manner in which the disease was located in colonial India – the fact that it was some sort of a disease, coupled with the speculative dimension connected to its causation. Second, how the reproduction of colonial knowledge/power about the 'irrational' and 'unscientific tribals' that have survived till today, amongst other things, form a part of the colonial and post-colonial 'civilizing mission' needs to be highlighted.

Various aspects of leprosy have been explored by scholars working on Europe, Africa, Australia, China, and India. Thus, Foucault refers to leprosy being seen along the logic of seclusion and control in the European world. We are told about 'treatment' methods in late medieval Europe that ranged from segregation to compulsory confinement of those affected by the disease.[2] In fact, government policy aimed to isolate and/or prosecute the leprosy-affected people, especially if they were Jews who were stereotyped and excluded as carriers of leprosy. Besides, the link between their 'insatiable sexual desire' – which made them susceptible to be carriers/transmitters of leprosy – does indeed appear to be a mind-boggling connection that drew upon the stereotyping of Jews.[3] Over the eighteenth century and early nineteenth century, the 'hereditary theory' of the disease that became popular in Europe perhaps reinforced some of these ideas. At the same time, the nineteenth century was also witnessing the shift towards bacteriology with its emphasis on the 'germ theory'. In fact, Hansen's discovery of the leprosy bacillus (*Mycobacterium leprae*) in 1873 needs to be contextualized keeping these features in mind.

'The empire strikes back'

The experience of the European world cannot be located in isolation during the latter half of the nineteenth century, which was marked by colonial expansion. In parts of colonial Africa – such as South Africa – stereotypes such as 'moral geography' and 'medical topography' were used as justification to exile and segregate certain groups of people who were affected by leprosy.[4] As can be perhaps expected, the location of the disease and its treatment assumed racist overtones. In colonial/semi-colonial China certain commonalities emerge, especially in the way disease was perceived, the stereotypes associated with those affected by it, the logic of segregation (which had pre-colonial origins), and the role of the missionaries.[5] The logic of seclusion and isolation determined the policy vis-à-vis those affected by the disease in Australia and New Zealand.[6] In these parts the church and the missionaries did play a prominent role.

Taken together, these reflected the anxieties of the colonialists in a period of colonial expansion, with the disease 'returning' as it were to haunt the world of metropolitan Europe. In fact, if anything the death of Father Damien, who worked in the leprosy colony of Molokai, Hawaii in 1889, only served to reinforce fears about the difficult-to-explain contagiousness of the disease in the colonies and in Britain.

It is in this overall global context that one needs to situate leprosy and explore its social history in colonial India while focusing on certain specificities. In fact, there has been a considerable amount of work on the social history of leprosy in colonial India.[7] Here one needs to highlight the pre/early colonial ideas related to the way in which the disease and those affected by it were located. However, as has already been mentioned, besides the use of Chaulmogra oil, the idea of isolating or confining those affected by it was not practised. In fact, those affected by leprosy were largely accommodated within society. And, if anything, the European experience of isolating and confining those suffering from the disease became a part of the policy practiced by the colonial state and its medical, legal, and administrative agencies in the period after Hansen's discovery (1873) and the post-Census operations (viz. 1869–1871). While Hansen had traced leprosy to the bacillus, the post-Census period quantified some statistical information about the number of people affected by the disease. This set into motion efforts to invisibilize the leprosy-affected and isolate/confine them as prisoners through the formulation of the Leprosy Acts. Thus, the leprosy affected were criminalized and not treated as those who were affected by a disease and needed care or treatment.

Consequently, what developed was nothing sort of a class offensive that was directed against the poor – which had clear racist overtones – leading to the arrest and forcible confinement of those affected by leprosy. After all, it was only the poor who could not 'hide' their disease either through their clothes or within the private spaces of their homes. Interestingly, the negotiations of the 'civilizing mission' with the disease were shaped by a set of speculative discourses, even as the Chaulmogra oil was adopted and used to comfort those affected by the disease.[8]

Historians working on leprosy in medieval Europe mention the idea of isolation/ forcible confinement as a practice affecting those who had leprosy (along with a host of other diseases), which in effect implied targeting the poor. As for the colonial medical establishment, India and its negotiations with the disease, besides the serious anxieties that have been already noted, these were shaped by the interaction of ideas and belief systems that originated from the metropolitan world of Europe of the nineteenth century and were projected as 'scientific' and 'progressive', along with the caste/class and gender-related notions of the colonial medical establishment and the emerging middle class, which were popularized through the (indigenous) print-culture.[9]

Here one has to bear in mind the existence of the poor ('pauper') lepers at pilgrimage sites such as Puri, which haunted the colonial imagination like a nightmare. Thus, over the nineteenth century, the colonial administration traced the source of the disease to centres of pilgrimage such as Puri. Leprosy seems to have received serious attention from the colonial authorities as early as 1874. The presence of those affected by the disease at Puri, which was identified as a major centre for leprosy – where they begged for alms and received charity during the annual congregation for the chariot festival associated with Jagannatha (viz. *ratha jatra*) – posed serious concerns for the colonial administration.

What is of course difficult to explain are the fears generated by leprosy in colonial Orissa if one considers the number of people affected by the disease (see Table 3.1). Thus, the *Census of 1871* quantified this data that comprised a miniscule section of the population.[10]

Table 3.1 Total number of lepers (1871)

Districts	Males	Females	Total
Cuttack	382	158	446 (0.298% of the population)
Balasore	177	17	194 (0.0252% -do-)
Puri	239	17	256 (0.0333% -do-)
Orissa Tributary states	160	21	181 (0.141% -do-)

Perhaps, one needs to factor in here the death of Father Damien, who worked in the leprosy colony of Molokai, Hawaii in 1889, which reinforced fears about this difficult-to-explain disease in Britain and its colonies and perhaps needs to be seen in terms of the 'empire striking back'.

Colonial 'unreason' and ways of explaining leprosy

The background years saw the most unscientific efforts that were prated as being 'scientific'. Journals associated with medical research also discussed the disease. One such article focused on Balasore, where a large amount of fish was consumed. Factors such as the age parameter (viz. that leprosy affected those between 15 and 40 years of age); the "fact" that it affected only males; the castes that were mostly affected (viz. the highest being agriculturalists); the "hereditary" nature of the disease (that invoked the Leprosy Report of the Royal College of Physicians), and under "certain conditions contagious"; fish consumption as a cause of the disease; and mostly fishermen as a "community" who were mostly affected by it.[11] As is clear, the focus was clearly on the poor – whether the agriculturists or the fisherfolk – who were affected by leprosy in Balasore.

Thus, it was the poverty of the leprosy affected that was a decisive factor that determined the manner in which the disease was located. The image of the 'semi naked' 'pauper lepers' who thronged and begged on the streets of Puri indeed made it easy to establish a direct connection between poverty and disease. After all, unlike the propertied sections, they could not hide their marks either by wearing clothes or by staying within the four walls of their domestic space. The logic associated with poverty was indeed profound and it was perhaps not a mere coincidence that the Naanka Durbikya – viz. the Famine of 1866 – was invoked as the starting point of it all. Thus, Stewart while compiling the details of Shaik Sheen Cowdse – an 18-year-old Muslim (Cuttack) – mentions how the disease 'commenced' after the 1866 Famine.[12] Though one can appreciate the possible effort to collect the evidence through some ways where he sought to get the details regarding the time when Cowdse got leprosy, it is also possible that a connection was being established between the disease and the Muslims. One has to also 'read' the description about Appee, a Chamar woman of 30 affected by the disease and who made and sold cheroots in Cuttack, in a similar manner.[13] Being a poor person's disease a Chamar woman could not, after all, escape getting leprosy. The reference to the "error of nutrition" such as the consumption of "unwholesome food", such as "stale or salted fish" – viz. *sukhua* – and "diseased" meat (beef?) was also seen as a cause of the disease.[14] What was overlooked was that *sukhua* was (and continues to be) a part of the plebeian diet along the coastal areas of Orissa, and also had serious connections with the process of preservation in a context (viz. nineteenth century) wherein refrigeration techniques did not exist. Thus, salt was mixed with the leftover catch that remained unsold and this was dried till it assumed the form of *sukhua* and sold later.

The consumption of beef by the Muslims who had 'unclean habits' was also expressed by Juggoo Mohun Roy as a cause of leprosy. Stewart added a comment, and as he put it, the Babu who "[was] a strict Hindu", to which he connected this viewpoint.[15] We are also told about leprosy being more common amongst Muslims than the Hindus – a point that was undoubtedly associated with beef consumption.[16] Interestingly, the question of 'heredity transmission' was discussed in connection with the well-to-do.[17]

Consequently, colonial interventions in Orissa provided a classic entry point to keep out the 'curse' of the disease and assert imperial superiority. It was tainted by racist, caste, and class hatred of the poor. This saw the enactment of the Leper's Act of 1898 that provided for the 'segregation' and medical treatment of 'pauper lepers'. Besides identifying it as a poor person's disease, the Act armed the colonial state to arrest and indeed to launch a class offensive against the poor. In fact, the Leper's Act III of 1898 – an all-India Act, introduced in 1901 to replace the Bengal Leper Act of 1895 – provided for the establishment of asylums to which "lepers may be sent from specified areas, for the arrest of pauper lepers found wandering in such areas, and for their detention in an asylum". It also empowered the local government to prohibit lepers from engaging in certain trades or occupations that were likely to endanger public health.[18]

Thus, people affected with leprosy were treated not as patients suffering from a disease but as prisoners. This logic became associated with a class offensive directed against the poor affected by leprosy formed the basis of colonial policy vis-à-vis leprosy. Consequently what can be clearly visualized is a context wherein a person affected by the disease was criminalized and arrested, instead of being located as a person suffering from a disease, who needed medical attention. In fact, the Magistrate of Puri and the President of Puri Leprosy House proposed a law to empower the Magistrate "to get any person of Pooree examined by the Civil Surgeon to ascertain whether he was suffering from the disease of leprosy". Those found to have leprosy were to be confined in a suitable asylum.[19]

As for the missionaries, the death of Father Damien (1889) was a rude shock since even though in the post-Hansen phase, the logic of leprosy's transmission and its cure were unknown. One can cite here James Risdon Bennett, *The Diseases of the Bible* (1887), as an example. This was reprinted at least twice after Father Damien's death (1889) and had a chapter on 'leprosy'.[20] The element of the 'empire striking back' was embedded in this exploration. Though this effort attempted to get back to the 'past', it was in fact very modern and was intended to explore the possibilities of working amongst those affected by leprosy. Supposedly a religious text, it transgresses the intended boundaries by incorporating the 'Western' medical systems that discussed leprosy. The fact that Bennett discusses India, almost at the outset of the section on leprosy, suggests the interactive component involving the metropolitan and the colonial world.[21] Without going into details one can also see how the colonial world and the disease is sought to be 'studied'. Whereas the tyrannical aspects of the past such as confinement and segregation are not discussed, the idea that the disease was brought back by those who went out on the 'crusades' is rejected and we are told that leprosy existed in the European continent prior to the 'crusades'. While delineating that it had affected the lower orders, he went on to argue that 'no class of society was exempt, not even royalty' from the disease. Nevertheless, the references to fish, salt deficiency, living conditions, habits, etc. are situated along with a note that "nothing has been definitely proved".[22] These co-exist with the idea of leprosy being contagious, the heredity factor, with both retaining a level of fluidity. Nevertheless, if seen holistically, this perhaps illustrates how the ideas of the missionaries in many ways echoed the point about leprosy's association with the poor, which perhaps provided the possibilities of working with the leprosy affected. The ideas related to leprosy's 'medieval' past appear to be rather 'modern' if seen together with the other factors, especially his support for segregation of the leprosy affected in the colonial world.[23] Finally, his basic effort was to help and encourage the missionary activities in the colonial world, and he commended the work of the "Mission of Lepers in India".[24] Thus, the "Mission of Lepers in India" seems to have been involved with Orissa from the early years of the twentieth century.[25]

The missionaries explained leprosy's causality as a disease of the soul, and also saw them work amongst those affected by the disease to provide them with relief. Thus, in practice they were more open-minded than the colonial establishment, even if the leprosy affected were confined to the 'homes' of the Mission.

Leprosy: the Adivasi healing systems and the Princely state of Keonjhar

Although 24 Princely states merged with Orissa during the process of decolonization, sources related to most them are indeed difficult to get access. After all, the darbars lacked any serious interest in this sector over the nineteenth century. Additionally, the diverse administrative structures to which the states were linked (viz. Central India, Bihar, Bengal, etc.) and the absence of preservation methods perhaps accounts for this problem. These factors perhaps account for the fact that the historiography related to the health systems in the Princely states of Orissa is yet to attract serious research.

This situation got somewhat altered over the twentieth century with local institutions associated with governance and the formation of the Orissa province in 1936, which strengthened this process. Some of the darbars did intervene in the sector of health also due to the threats posed by some diseases such as leprosy and smallpox, as well as the ideas of improving their governance. Here the pressures of the colonial health establishment, the local government, and the indirect effect of the state peoples' movement from the mid-1930s need to be factored in. After all, sectors such as health (and education, etc.) were areas where the Congress Ministry (1937–1939), the local government, and the colonial agencies were willing to spend some resources.[26]

Before examining the two Princely states of Keonjhar and Mayurbhanj, it needs to be delineated that the idea of confining the leprosy affected led to the construction of the Cuttack Leprosy Asylum in 1919. This had certain implications for the Princely states. Thus, the colonial medical and legal establishment were involved in a decision that included the Princely states from where the leprosy affected could be sent to the Cuttack Leprosy Asylum.[27] Of course, as would be seen, both Keonjhar and Mayurbhanj had their own Leprosy Asylums.

At the very outset we had mentioned the ideas of the Adivasis about evil spirits causing leprosy. The Gadbas, for example, linked the disease to the *duma* (ghost) of a god.[28] Nevertheless, the logic of the diversities and the deeper nuances need to be highlighted. Here one needs to highlight how the Santals for example located the treatment of leprosy. Bodding's description of the 'treatment' included medicine that was a combination of seeds, fruits, parts of birds, etc. that had to be cooked and eaten, along with anointing the body of the person affected by leprosy with red lead and other ingredients – including oil – every day. A major component included abstinence from sexual intercourse, meat and fish, and alcoholic drinks. Specific details outlined the method to anoint sores with a preparation that contained amongst other things melted butter from cow's milk. The 'treatment' included baths and washing of the hands.[29] What seems particularly striking is a level of Hinduization – with its stress on vegetarianism and abstinence from alcohol and sexual intercourse – though the actual composition of the medicine does seem contradictory. Of course, what needs emphasis is that beyond the stereotyping of the Adivasi world in terms of witchcraft and sorcery, there were healers with specific 'prescriptions' for specific diseases.

As for the Princely state of Keonjhar, its negotiations with leprosy seem to be rather interesting, especially when it comes to certain common meeting points with the Santal system of 'treatment'. Both appear to be in striking contrast to the colonial policy of segregation and confinement. Our discussion on Keonjhar is based on the palm-leaf manuscripts preserved by the descendants of the erstwhile ruling family of Keonjhar and the popular oral traditions.[30] Although these palm-leaf manuscripts describe several aspects related to treating leprosy in Keonjhar since the seventeenth century, one needs to be careful about its 'origins', given the search for 'ancientness' of most of the Princely states and their rulers in colonial Orissa This was associated with the very process of securing legitimacy from the colonial power and saw a virtual competition amongst the different Princely states of Orissa, who sought to prove their 'ancientness'. In fact, one would venture to even argue that they were most probably produced only in the nineteenth century.[31]

The palm-leaf manuscripts and the popular oral tradition suggest that one of the kings, who ruled before the seventeenth century, had learnt in a dream about the usefulness of the Bhramaramari plant as a cure for leprosy. Furthermore, he was 'advised' to popularize the plant for the welfare of the people. The Raja (king) in fact looked upon this dream as a divine intervention – a theme that is stressed by references to the popular oral tradition. In the dream, the king was ordered to locate the plant at a specific site in the dense forest. He was given detailed instructions regarding the method of using it for the treatment of leprosy. This dream became the basis for a process associated with the virtual deification of the plant and its subsequent ascendancy to the position of a local deity in the region. Subsequently, the royal order of Keonjhar employed a priestly class called *dehuri* for the worship of the Bhramaramari plant in the woods. The *dehuri* enjoyed certain privileges and was also entrusted with the responsibility of collecting parts of the Bhramaramari plant, which were handed over to the Raja of Keonjhar.

According to the oral tradition, the Bhramaramari plant was originally available around a forest-ridden village called Kuntala in Keonjhar. It was also believed that its medicinal qualities developed with the ripening of the trunk. Its name (Bhramaramari) was derived from the wandering beetles, which met their death when they came into contact with the plant. Hence the name Bhramaramari came to mean the killing of beetles (bhramara = beetles; mari = to kill). Perhaps the death of a large number of beetles that happened to fly over the plant spurred the imagination of the Adivasi folk to name it this way. In their perception, the plant itself emerged as a centre of divinity – a goddess possessing healing qualities.[32]

The small branches of the Bhramaramari plant, received from the *dehuri*, was preserved in the royal storehouse known as Bhramaramari Bhandara (storehouse), under the supervision of a royal officer called Gantayita. Leprosy patients from different parts of the state and outside thronged the gate of the palace with the hope of getting the Bhramaramari medicine. They openly assembled at the palace without any fear of the stigma attached to leprosy. The medicine was given to leprosy patients with detailed instructions regarding the method of using it. However, with the growth of print-culture, a leaflet containing the instructions called *Byabastha Patra* ('Information regarding the use of medicine') was also supplied to each patient, along with the medicine. The king distributed this medicine personally, free of cost to the patients at his doorstep, as the principal devotee of the goddess. From the point of view of his own people, this enabled him to demonstrate his charitable inclination, through which he could assert his position as their chief.

The palm-leaf manuscripts provide details explaining the use of Bhramaramari medicine to the patients. They list the various spices, leaves and portions of the plant which were to be dried and ground. These ingredients had to be converted into paste and the prescribed quantity applied (twice daily) by the leprosy patients. The patients were instructed "not to see the face of women" and to avoid non-vegetarian food, milk, and anything that was sour or sweet. They were advised to avoid massages while bathing. More significantly, the instructions also stressed that the patients should remain isolated in a room. The prescribed diet included hot rice, dried salt, and *kalara* (viz. bitter gourd) leaves which have a bitter taste, etc. and emphasized the use of warm and boiled water. After remaining isolated over a period of one to three weeks, the patients were expected to come out and offer *bhog* and *puja* to Shiva and Balabhadra, the state deities of Keonjhar. Hence both these gods had to be finally approached for their blessings in order to get cured.

The dietary prescription, with its stress on vegetarianism, demonstrate a significant level of Hinduization. The stress on warm and boiled water seems particularly striking and perhaps reflects the interaction with the colonial medical system. The idea that 'male' patients should not see the 'face of women' illustrates the importance given to male patients when it comes to the availability of the treatment. This also raises a question if this 'treatment' was for women at all. Besides, it also suggests a level of sexual restraint that seems to have been prescribed. Although the importance attached to segregation and enforce sexual restraint can be read as a pointer to the process of Hinduization itself, it is worth speculating if it had anything to do with an awareness that human contact could spread leprosy. In a context that witnessed the segregation and arrest of those affected by disease, the logic of this 'liberalism' – independent of the 'treatment' of the disease – seems to be particularly striking.

As seen, there were deeper and complex implications that sustained this drive from the point of view of the darbar. Thus, a social historian of health and medicine needs to see this as a process related to the feudal order's search for legitimacy in the crisis-ridden phase of the nineteenth century. One needs to for example refer to the Famine of 1866 – the Naanka Durbikhya – which, as received wisdom suggests, devastated the coastal tract comprising Cuttack, Puri, and Balasore. However new research suggests that the entire region including the Princely states and the Chotanagpur tract were devastated by it. The level of variation in terms of its impact on human life was primarily due to the alternative food systems in the Western 'interior' tract.[33] The Keonjhar darbar's initiatives in this sense seem to go beyond accepting leprosy as a disease, as it provided space for its 'treatment' through what was to become a formal, ritualized affair and got to settle people affected by the Famine – including those affected by leprosy, or those excommunicated, since they had accepted food from the colonial relief system.

In fact, one needs to perhaps see the annual congregations in the context of the lack of possible alternatives as well. As reported, it was difficult to get "competent" medical personnel and the darbar had to manage with "a partially qualified medical assistant" who had studied in the Cuttack Medical College.[34] We are told that this was the only medical officer in the Killah (viz. castle town). This difficulty was attributed to the inaccessibility of the Princely state.[35] In many ways this illustrates how the Princely state of Keonjhar had no serious interest when it came to investment in the health sector.

The response of the colonial medical establishment over the closing years of the nineteenth century seems particularly striking. Thus, in a context wherein the cure for leprosy was unavailable, the basic ideas about it remained unchanged and its speculative discourses continued. Thus, even in the early years of the twentieth century, J.T. Calvert expressed his anxiety about the leprosy-affected people moving around and mixing freely in the initial phase of getting the disease. He was categorical about it being "hereditary" and the poor "unclean" people helping its "progress". He speculated about the "fish theory", that "cannot be proved". What is rather significant is his point that the municipal bodies in "any part of the district" were yet to take any step to "segregate the lepers or to treat the disease". In many ways then this position echoed a level of disinterest and matches with the notion of the disease being "God's curse": It expressed a level of unconcern about a disease that clearly affected only a very microscopic section of the population, especially the poor.[36] Puri – the 'pilgrim centre' – was supposed to be more "tainted", at least in the speculative discourses of the early years of the twentieth century. Besides mentioning that the leprosy affected were very "visible", E.E. Waters mentioned that "lepers are not admitted in the dispensaries of this district", and since they received charity they were "not likely to come into the hospital books". He continued with the argument about the "lower class Uriyas" being a "dirty race" who had no ideas about cleanliness or sanitation being the storehouse of the disease. His reference to the "putrid fish theory" and its connection with leprosy was contradictory, given the speculative nature of colonial medical discourse that was supposedly based on 'observations'. Thus, he invoked the observations made at the Satpara and the Banpur dispensary. The former was located in the Chilka area – which exported large amounts of "cured fish" – where leprosy was "uncommon". However, the Banpur dispensary, which was close by, "show[ed] a disproportionately large number of leprosy cases".[37]

The anti-imperialist struggle – especially the Gandhian ideals related to working amongst those affected by leprosy – did generate a marginal shift in the way people located those affected by the disease. Nevertheless, the policy of 'non-intervention' in the affairs of the Princely states – a policy advocated by Gandhi and adopted by the Congress, perhaps accounted for the lack of any serious political initiatives, which meant continuities in the way the leprosy affected were perceived in the Princely states.

The formation of the province of Orissa (1936) and the popular ministry (in 1937) seem to have led to the evolution of a policy on leprosy. Thus, a three-pronged strategy was developed to negotiate leprosy. This included isolation, treatment, and propaganda that suggest distinct continuities.[38] The propaganda component was taken very seriously and 20,000 leaflets were printed in 1938 in different languages and circulated in the province.[39] The three-pronged strategy was based on mundane and speculative ideas that upheld confinement and hardly impacted any change as far as the leprosy affected were concerned. Nevertheless, these seemed to trigger some activity in the Princely states.

As for Keonjhar, the 1931 Census marked out 69:100,000 people who were affected by leprosy, which was a very small part of the population of the state.[40] The reference to the recruitment of a new compounder "trained in the treatment of leprosy" for the Anandapur clinic in Keonjhar matches the way in which such reports were usually drafted.[41] However, the point about the treatment needs to be qualified since the disease was yet to be fully curable and needs to be seen in the context of the widespread use of Chaulmogra oil. There were two leprosy clinics in the state, where 1856 injections were administered – viz. at Anandapur 1664 and at Soso 192.[42] One is not clear about these injections. Most probably it was Chaulmogra oil that was injected and one can perhaps see in this 'Mr Science' being tamed by the 'irrational' and 'unscientific' world of 'magic' and 'superstition' in colonial India.

The Princely state of Keonjhar seems to have taken the propaganda aspect against leprosy rather seriously. Thus, in 1939–1940, a leprosy 'propaganda officer' was appointed and the sub-assistant surgeon of Telkir was sent to the Tropical School of Medicine, Calcutta for training in leprosy treatment. There was a decline in the number of people who were injected (viz. 1370 in 1939–1940), which was attributed to the 'impatience' of the patients to the prolonged treatment. The darbar also intensified the surveys in the state to detect the leprosy-affected people.[43] Although not spelt out, the logic of these surveys was to search for the leprosy affected so as to segregate and confine them in the Leprosy Asylums of the State that stigmatized those affected by the disease, who were not comfortable with it.

The reports demonstrated the self-congratulatory attitude of the darbar in its negotiations with leprosy. What seems to have been overlooked is the absence of a serious way in which the state people could perceive that they were being actually cured of the disease, even after going through the painful process of being injected. Consequently, the effort to highlight the increase in the number of those injected (viz. to 2080 in 1940–1941) was nothing more than harping on and highlighting the statistical dimension.[44]

Mayurbhanj

Missionary interventions in Orissa associated with leprosy began in Mayurbhanj in 1879, when the Roman Catholic Mission, which was also known as the Nagalkata (a village) Mission was founded. Later on Krishnachandrapur, a village formed out of clearing a portion of the jungle and named after the king Krishna Chandra Bhanj Deo who had donated the land, became the centre on the Roman Catholic Mission.[45]

'The Mission of Lepers' extended "generous" help to the Leper Asylum at Baripada. In 1929 it had 100 inmates, out of whom eight were "dismissed", 11 died, and 81 inmates lived in the Asylum by the end of the year. Miss Charles was in charge of this Asylum. It seems to have been realized that it was risky to have small children – most probably accompanying their parents – living too close to the leprosy quarters. Hence, there was a proposal for building "new" and "suitable quarters" for the leprosy affected.[46] It is possible that that this "realization" in some ways questioned the hereditary factors associated with leprosy, in a context wherein the 'germ theory' of disease had gained a serious acceptance in the metropolitan and the colonial medical establishment.

The details related to the number of the leprosy affected stood at 79 per 100,000 of population in 1931 in the state, and we are told that the numbers had "more than doubled" since the 1911 Census. In 1931 the number of the leprosy affected stood at 708 (453 males and 255 females) in the state. The stigma associated with the disease made the relatives conceal it in case they approached 'marriageable age'.[47] Out of the total number of affected people amongst the Christians in the State Leper Asylum at Baripada, 58 were 'lepers', which the Census Officer felt was "difficult to accept" – thereby almost privileging the 'master race'. Keen to resolve the matter he mentioned how those who were admitted into the asylum had adopted Christianity as "their management was in the hands of the missionaries of the Evangelical Society".[48] We are told about the inmates being treated twice a week by the staff of the Leper Clinic. The state launched an anti-leprosy campaign in September 1930 under the charge of a Special Officer who had been trained in the School of Tropical Medicine in Calcutta.[49] The details of these campaigns are not mentioned. Nevertheless, they seem to be guided by speculative discourses in a context when treatment methods were not known to the colonial health establishment. Of course, the manner in which the conditions of the Adivasis in the 'interior' were described perhaps illustrates the way the darbar located the disease and the people in the margins. Thus, in 1924–1925 we are told about the 'aboriginals' having better health.[50] Similarly, Bamanaghati which was a predominantly Adivasi tract, was supposed to be 'relatively immune' to leprosy.[51] Such articulations were like justifications of the darbar's disinterest in the 'interior' areas inhabited by the socially excluded Adivasis and outcastes/low castes when it comes to interventions related to health.

The Mayurbhanj health system was Baripada-centric as is clear from the reports. The *Administrative Report of 1935–36* mentions two *kutcha* sheds that had been constructed to 'treat' leprosy patients in the dispensaries at Bangripsi and Udala. The state attached a lot of importance to the anti-leprosy campaign and five clinics were assigned to oversee this task. Moreover it conducted "thorough home to home" surveys to catch and confine the leprosy-affected to the Leprosy Asylums. The Leper Asylum at Baripada had 132 inmates (as against 98 cases the year before) and 65 were described as "cases under special treatment". Operations were also conducted on the leprosy patients, most probably by Dr Maheshwar Pati M.B. the Assistant Surgeon. Some of the details mentioned illustrate certain "hidden" features. Thus, five of the inmates had been "arrested"; nine were "quiescent" (presumably quiet/inactive); and four of them "ran away". The reference to the inmates "occupying the verandah" indicates how the Asylum was over-crowded. We are told about the inmates "beautifying" their surrounding – with a silence on how the labour for this was ensured – along with the need for more water. The report acknowledged the support of "Christian friends in England and other places" who provided funds, clothing, and books.[52]

The *Administrative Report of 1941–42* mentions that the police stations covering Rairanpur, Bahalda, Besai, Betnoti, Baisinga, Udla, Baripada, and Muruda were surveyed to detect "leprosy cases". Not only were 32 villages surveyed, but 419 villages were re-surveyed with a force comprising 15 people ranging from a leprosy officer and a Sub-Assistant Surgeon, compounders, leprosy workers, peons, and sweepers. This led to the "detection" of 211 leprosy-affected people, most of whom were "aboriginal classes". The report mentions the presence of 126 inmates in the Baripada Leprosy Asylum. These included some inmates who had been "arrested" with "deformity", whose condition was stated to be "worse" than the others. During the year three "young lads" were "discharged with certificates".[53]

Conclusion

We began by outlining a range of diversities including leprosy's 'past' to explore the way it was located and negotiated in different geographical spaces and contexts. The changes related to the manner in which the disease was perceived, including the fears and insecurities it generated in the age of colonial expansion, have been highlighted. These were marked by serious shifts and changes in the way leprosy was sited in the latter half of the nineteenth century. Proceeding further, we delineated how the colonial medical establishment and 'Mr Science' sought to engage with leprosy to uphold the 'civilizing mission' in India. What we have outlined clearly shows the speculative, unscientific, and irrational ideas that had broad interactional foundations between the metropolitan world and the colonial medical establishment, as well as sections of the Oriya middle class, which legitimized it.

This chapter also examined the Adivasi methods related to the treatment of leprosy. Additionally, we have explored the negotiations of Keonjhar and Mayurbhanj with the disease. The shift – especially when it comes to the Keonjhar darbar's engagement with leprosy over the nineteenth and the twentieth century along with that of Mayurbhanj over the latter phase – shows the distinct footprints of the colonial order's policies of targeting of the poor through arrests, segregation, and confinement in the two Princely states. Thus, the darbar retreated to a position that Jane Buckingham had critiqued in her study of leprosy in colonial south India which had located the leprosy affected as prisoners and not as people who were ill.[54]

Our sources are silent about the leprosy-affected people who were confined in the Princely states of Orissa. This is rather striking and this prevents a social historian from grappling with the problems faced by these sections, unlike in different parts of colonial India. Thus, Sanjeev Kakar refers to the leprosy affected during the nineteenth century detesting their confinement that reduced them to "prisoners" in cases where they were forcibly confined. He refers to the emulation of medieval European methods of sexual segregation that was practised by the colonial health establishment which was also hated. Kakar mentions certain noticeable shifts over the twentieth century. Thus in 1939 there was a "Lepers strike in Cochin" and two leprosy-affected youths sat on a hunger strike demanding admission to the Asylum at Adoor.[55] Similarly in colonial Orissa there is evidence of different forms of protest by the inmates of the Asylum at Cuttack (that had been established in 1919). Issues ranging from the pain and unhappiness, the purposeless logic of being in the Asylum (perhaps since the disease was attributed to one's fate), to witnessing the people who had advance stages of leprosy die in the 1920s made many inmates escape from the Asylum. In 1940 the method of treatment, the fear of the injections, and the quality of rice provided saw the first strike by the inmates in the Asylum.[56] Beginning with a phase when the Princely states did not put in records related to health, this silence on the confined can be perhaps attributed to the despotic order in these enclaves.

We are told about how the discovery of Promin, a sulfone drug in 1941, was shown to successfully cure leprosy.[57] However, nothing remarkable seems to have got altered in the Princely states till India's Independence, and leprosy continues to haunt the imagination of the people in a free country, even up to the present times.[58] How else does one explain the Ranchi district administration permitting leprosy patients who were denied rations for months for "lacking fingers and thumbs for biometric verification" to finally collect it on 14 September 2016? Ranchi is the capital of Jharkhand, and as is well known, it has a large Adivasi and Low-Caste/Dalit population.[59]

Notes

1 'World's First Leprosy Vaccine, From Indian Lab, to Go on Trial', *Times of India*, 21 August 2016, http://timesofindia.indiatimes.com/city/chennai/Worlds-first-leprosy-vaccine-from-Indian-lab-to-go-on-trial/articleshow/53791544.cms (accessed on 12 January 2017).

2   Michael Foucault, *Madness and Civilisation: A History of Insanity in the Age of Reason*, Vintage: New York, 1988, 1–5.
3   For details, Sheldon Watts, *Epidemics and History: Disease, Power and Imperialism*, London: Yale University Press, 1997, 44–64.
4   Harriet Deacon, 'Racial Segregation and Medical Discourse in Nineteenth Century Cape Town', *Journal of South African Studies*, 22(2), 1996, 287–308.
5   Angela Ki Che Leung, *Leprosy in China: A History*, New York: Columbia University Press, 2009.
6   For details see Rod Edmond, *Leprosy and Empire: A Medical and Cultural History*, Cambridge: Cambridge University Press, 2007.
7   The pioneers in this field have been Sanjiv Kakkar, *The Patient, the Person: Empowering the Leprosy Patient*, New Delhi: Danlep, 1992; 'Leprosy in British India, 1860–1940; Colonial Politics and Missionary Medicine', *Medical History*, 40(2), 1996, 215–30; 'Leprosy in India; The Intervention of Oral History', *Oral History*, 23(1), 1995, 37–45; and 'Medical Developments and Patient Unrest in the Leprosy Asylum' in Biswamoy Pati and Mark Harrison (ed.), *Health, Medicine and Empire: Perspectives on Colonial India*, Delhi: Orient Longman, 2001, 188–216; and Jane Buckingham, *Leprosy in Colonial South India: Medicine and Confinement*, Basingstoke: Palgrave, 2002. Shubhada Pandya, '"Regularly Brought up Medical Men": Nineteenth-century Grant Medical College Graduates, Medical Rationalism and Leprosy', *Indian Economic and Social History Review*, 41(3), 2004, 293–314, discusses Indian medical students and the way they located leprosy. See also James Staples, *Peculiar People, Amazing Lives: Leprosy, Social exclusion and Community Making in South India*, Delhi: Orient Longman, 2007, which provides valuable contemporary insights. Manmohan Krishna, 'The Social History of Leprosy in Colonial Bihar and Chotanagpur, 1870s-1940s', Engages With the Complexities of the Disease; M.Phil. Dissertation, Delhi University, 2012.
8   There is a reference to experimenting with Gurjan oil on the leprosy-affected convicts at the Andamans – Home Dep./Port Blair Br. Nos. 19–22 A, October 1873, National Archives of India (hereafter NAI).
9   For details Biswamoy Pati and Chandi P. Nanda, 'The Leprosy Patient and Society: Colonial Orissa, 1870s – 1940s', in Biswamoy Pati and Mark Harrison (eds.), *The Social History of Health and Medicine in Colonial India*, London: Routledge, 2009, 113–28.
10 W.W. Hunter, *A Statistical Account of Bengal: Districts of Cuttack and Balasore*, Vol. XVIII, London: Trubner & Co., 1877, 67, 267; W.W. Hunter, *A Statistical Account of Bengal: Districts of Puri and the Orissa Tributary States, London*, Vol. XIX, London: Trubner & Co, 1877, 30, 208.
11 Vincent Richards, Civil Surgeon, Balasore, 'Statistical Notes on Leprosy in Northern Orissa', *Indian Annals of Medical Science*, XVI, 1873–74, 303–18.
12 'Distribution and Causation of Leprosy in British India, 1875', W.D. Stewart, Civil Surgeon, Cuttack, 24 March 1877, 45, National Library of Scotland (hereafter NLS). http://digital.nls.uk/indiapapers/browse/pageturner.cfm?id=74506472&mode=transcription (accessed on 20 September 2016).
13 Stewart, 43, NLS.
14 Stewart, to the Deputy Surgeon General Presidency Circle, 21 March, 1877, even as it argued about leprosy being 'confined chiefly to the poorer classes', 42, NLS.
15 J.M. Roy, Cuttack, 17 March 1877, in Stewart, 46, NLS.
16 From Babu Kedarnath Panday, Native Doctor to the Civil Surgeon Midnapur, 10 March 1877; Pandey was discussing this in the context of the district of Moorshedabad, NLS.
17 Keshab Chundra Mukherjee, Native Doctor in charge of Golegram Charitable Dispensary to the Civil Surgeon of Midnapur, Memorandum no. 6, 23 February 1877, 12, NLS.
18 L.S.S. O'Malley, *Census of India, 1911, Volume V, Bengal, Bihar and Orissa and Sikkim, Part I, Report*, Calcutta: Bengal Secretariat Book Depot, 1913, 425.

19 Joseph Armstrong, acting magistrate and president, Pooree Leprosy House Committee, in his proposal to the commissioner of Orissa, Accession Number 39792, Board of Revenue, Secretariat Records (loose), Orissa State Archives.

20 James Risdon Bennett, *The Diseases of the Bible*, London: Religious Tract Society, 1887. This was reprinted in 1891 and 1896, Chapter 1, 15–55.

21 Bennett, *The Diseases*, 18.

22 *Ibid.*, 27.

23 *Ibid.*, 54–5.

24 *Ibid.*, 54.

25 For details, Mission to Lepers in India and the Far East (founded in 1874), *Twentieth Annual Report for the Year 1894*, London: John F. Shaw, 10–11, lists where it operated in India.

26 For details K.M. Patra, *Orissa State Legislature and Freedom Struggle: 1912–47*, New Delhi: Peoples Publishing House, 1979; without going into details, the Private Papers related to some of the Princely states (at the NMML, New Delhi) illustrate this point.

27 Home Dep./Medical Br., Proceedings nos. 15, Part B, October 1919, NAI.

28 Verrier Elwin, *Tribal Myths of Orissa*, London: Oxford University Press, 1954, 487.

29 Rev. P.O. Bodding, *Studies in Santal Medicine and Connected Folklore*, Calcutta: The Asiatic Society, 2011 (originally published in 1925–40), 255–6.

30 M.M. Mishra, 'A Note on Leprosy: Sources Based on the Palm-leaf Manuscripts of the Rajasabha of the Erstwhile Keonjhar State', Oriya, unpublished. These manuscripts represent what can be perhaps seen as a shift from an oral to a written tradition. I acknowledge C.P. Nanda's help in procuring this source material; for details also see Pati and Nanda, 'The Leprosy Patient and Society', 113–15.

31 Details related to this 'competition' is delineated in 'The Brief Histories of Each of the 24 States (1909)', R/2 (285/1), Crown Representative Papers, India Office Library, London.

32 According to the oral tradition, the Bhramaramari plant was originally available around a forest-ridden village called Kuntala in Keonjhar. It was also believed that its medicinal qualities developed with the ripening of the trunk. Its name (Bhramaramari) was derived from the wandering beetles which met their death when they came into contact with the plant. Hence the name Bhramaramari came to mean the killing of beetles (bhramara = beetles; mari = to kill). Perhaps the death of a large number of beetles that happened to fly over the plant spurred the imagination of the Adivasi folk to name it this way. In their perception, the plant itself emerged as a centre of divinity – a goddess possessing healing qualities.

33 For details, Biswamoy Pati, 'Beyond Geographical Boundaries: Chotanagpur and North-Western Orissa, 1850s-1930', and Vinita Damodaran, 'Towards an Environmental History of Chotanagpur: The Land and the Forests of Chotanagpur in the Nineteenth Century', in Lata Singh and Biswamoy Pati (eds.), *Colonial and Contemporary Bihar and Jharkhand*, New Delhi: Primus, 2014, 9–28 and 59–90, respectively.

34 Home Department / Medical Branch, Proceedings 5–7, July 1894, NAI.

35 Home Dep. / Medical Br., Proc. 5–7, July 1894, NAI, From the Government Agent of Keonjhar to the Superintendent of Tributary Mahals, Cuttack, 2 February 1894.

36 Major J.T. Calvert, IMS, Civil Surgeon, Cuttack, to the Inspector General of Civil Hospitals, Bengal, No. 459, 21 March 1904, Government of Bengal, Municipal Dep./ Medical Br., May 1904.

37 Captain E.E. Waters, MD, Civil Surgeon Puri to Inspector General Hospitals of Civil Hospitals, Bengal, No. 261, 30 March 1904, Government of Bengal, Municipal Dep./ Medical Br.

38 G. Verghese, *Annual Public Health Report of the Province of Orissa for the Year 1937 and the Vaccination Report for the Year 1937–38*, Cuttack: Orissa Government Press, 1939, 24.

39 G. Verghese, *Annual Public Health Report of the Province of Orissa for the year 1938 and the Vaccination Report for the year 1938–39*, Cuttack: Government Press, 1940, 40.

40 M. Laeequddin, Census Officer, *Census of Mayurbhanj, Vol. 1*, Calcutta: Caledonian Printing Co., 1937, in fact, discussed the details related to the number of leprosy-affected people in some of the Princely states. As mentioned, Athgarh had the highest – 144 leprosy-affected people per 100,000 people, and Bamra the lowest number of people affected by the disease – 43:100,000; of course Puri had the highest number of people affected by the disease in the Province as well as the states – 155:100,00; 223.

41 *Annual Report on the Administration of the Keonjhar State for 1937–38*, Keonjhargarh: Keonjhar State Press, 1939, 41.

42 *Annual Report on the Administration of the Keonjhar State for 1938–39*, Keonjhargarh: Keonjhar State Press, 1940, 44.

43 *Annual Report on the Administration of the Keonjhar State for 1939–40*, Keonjhargarh: Keonjhar State Press, 1942, 45; 47.

44 *Annual Report on the Administration of the Keonjhar State for 1940–41*, Keonjhargarh: Keonjhar State Press, 1942, 41.

45 Mohammad Laeequddin, Census Officer, *Census of Mayurbhanj State Vol. I, 1931*, Calcutta: Caledonian Printing Co., 1937, 132.

46 *Report on the Administration of Mayurbhanj 1929–30*, Baripada: State Press Mayurbhanj, 1930, 104.

47 Laeequddin, *Census of Mayurbhanj State Vol. I*, 223–4.

48 *Ibid.*, 225; 228.

49 *Ibid.*, 227.

50 *Report on the Administration of Mayurbhanj 1924–25*, Baripada: State Press Mayurbhanj, 1925, 70.

51 Laeequddin, *Census of Mayurbhanj State Vol. I*, 227–8.

52 *Report on the Administration of Mayurbhanj 1935–36*, Baripada: State Press Mayurbhanj, 1939, 81. Dr Pati performed surgical operations that ranged from radical mastoid and cataract to sarcoma and cancer. The Baripada Hospital had an X-Ray machine. There was a female hospital at Baripada along with a lady doctor S.B. Santra. Moreover, there was a Medical Library that had journals such as the *IMG*, *The Calcutta Medical Journal*, and the *International Medical Digest* and books that were supposed to "Keep up Professional Knowledge", 69, 71–2, 74, 77, 109–10.

53 *Report on the Administration of Mayurbhanj 1941–42*, Baripada: State Press Mayurbhanj, 1944, 101–2.

54 Buckingham, *Leprosy in Colonial South India*.

55 S. Kakkar, 'Medical Developments and Patient Unrest in the Leprosy Asylum' in Biswamoy Pati and Mark Harrison (eds.), *Health, Medicine and Empire: Perspectives on Colonial India*, New Delhi: Orient Longman, 2001, 188–216.

56 Pati and Nanda, 'The Leprosy Patient and Society', 120–3.

57 These details are taken from www.niaid.nih.gov/topics/leprosy/understanding/Pages/history.aspx (accessed on 6 September 2016).

58 And moving beyond imagination, according to the estimates of the National Leprosy Eradication Programme, about 1 lakh leprosy-affected people have been detected every year since 2005 – the year the WHO declared India to be leprosy-free. Besides, 1.27 lakh new cases were detected in 2013–2014; for details http://nlep.nic.in

59 'Ration and Relief for Leprosy Patients', *The Telegraph*, 15 September 2016, www.telegraphindia.com/1160915/jsp/frontpage/story_108288.jsp#.V9unQkma2X2 – (accessed on 16 September 2016).

4 Smallpox in the Princely enclaves of Orissa

In a place 25% of the people died of smallpox and 3,600 are now alive; what was the population of that country?[1]

The above question from a mathematics textbook in Oriya of the 1870s perhaps defines smallpox that was undoubtedly a dreaded disease that was caused by the variola virus. This chapter explores certain complexities associated with smallpox in some of the Princely states of Orissa. In a broader context certain aspects related to the disease need to be delineated, especially the pre-vaccine phase of human survival against smallpox. Here one needs to refer to variolation or inoculation which was the method first used to immunize an individual against smallpox (Variola) with material taken from a patient or a recently variolated individual so that a mild, but protective infection, resulted.

As for China, disagreeing with J. Needham who traces the practice of variolation to the tenth century, Angela K.C. Leung mentions that the first reliable practice of variolation against smallpox is documented in the seventeenth-century records. Discussing the details of variolation, Leung outlines three methods of variolation. The first method involved putting in a piece of cotton imbued with pox pus into the nostril of the healthy child; the second involved using a squama when a fresh pustule was not available; the third method involved making a healthy child wear the clothes of a child who had contracted the disease. Exposed to any of these methods meant that the child got fever for seven days after which the process of variolation was completed. Leung mentions that the vaccine was first introduced in Macau, after which it reached Canton around 1805.[2]

We get references to the method of variolation practiced in different parts of Africa. Thus "the pox was pricked with a thorn, saved on a plantain leaf and then rubbed into the scratched area of a healthy person's arm."[3] Scholars also mention African slave sources that referred to the prevalence of this practice in parts of Africa as well.[4]

Harve Bazin refers to the method of inoculation reaching the European world from Turkey, where the inoculators were mostly women. Lady Mary Wortley Montagu is credited not only for her observations about the method in Turkey, where her husband was posted as the British Ambassador to the Ottoman empire in Constantinople (between 1716–1718), but also 'carrying' this method to England. She returned in 1721 to London, when a smallpox epidemic had hit England and got her three-year-old daughter inoculated. Bazin refers to the first wave of inoculation in England over the years 1722–1730, and this being adopted in the continent as well.[5]

As for colonial India, David Arnold has been a pioneer when it comes to research on the social history of smallpox.[6] At the same time, there has been a shift towards region-based studies that unravel the specificities and diversities of South Asia. Thus, for regions such as Orissa, Madras, and Goa,[7] the 'resistance' to smallpox vaccination and a host of other complexities have attracted a lot of scholarly attention.[8] A part of the 'civilizing mission', the colonial vaccination policy has also led to studies on the technological aspects and government policy.[9] Nevertheless, the Princely states have been a relatively ignored area when it comes to scholarly research related to smallpox – a point that has been already mentioned in the chapter on leprosy.

The attempt in this chapter is to take up some of the Princely states of Orissa and explore smallpox against a canvas of social history. I do not see 'indigenous' cultures as autonomously generating their own ideas, notions, and solutions, independent of the non-tribal communities and colonialism.[10] Instead, I accept interactions amongst them and highlight areas of contestations and resistance, as well as the acceptance of the colonial power/knowledge system. One needs to be particularly sensitive to the phenomenon of Hinduization of tribal communities while working on this area. It was through this process that the Adivasis were sought to be 'integrated' with Hindu (caste) society in order to exploit and exercise power over them. From the point of view of the Adivasis, Hinduization implied an acceptance as well as a rejection of various features of non-tribal, Hindu society. This co-existed with a contestatory aspect vis-à-vis the Oriya (non-tribal) community. Alongside some specific elements of the non-tribal groups, including certain practices such as inoculation, 'black magic' and the so-called subversive cults demonstrate the close affinities some of these had with the tribal communities. A point that needs to be emphasized here is that the tribal world cannot be territorialized in terms of the boundaries of the Princely states and the Orissa Districts, or subsequently the Orissa Province.

Smallpox and the world of the tribals

The colonization of Orissa inaugurated many shifts and changes which were reflected in various ways, including the manner in which the tribal communities related to health, disease, and medicine, including smallpox. The tribal communities had (and still have) an oral tradition that offer us fascinating clues to their vision and worldviews of health, disease, and medicine. That health was considered extremely vital is reflected in the importance attached to the medicine men and women which not only illustrates a constant battle with certain forces, but also the necessity of a virtual 'specialist'.

How did the tribal population locate smallpox? Nothing specific can be cited here, though the discourse of colonial officials and bureaucrats offers mono-dimensional explanations, often associated with the world of magic, spirits, and ghosts.[11] Such constructions appear to ignore the philosophies of disease and instead project the stereotypical image of the 'irrational' and 'unscientific' tribal. What is rarely mentioned in these discourses is an underlying set of inter-connections between the colonial military inroads that were unleashed on the tribal world, smallpox, and the negotiations that they entailed.[12] One can see this is the case of the tribal population of western Orissa.

Coming to the tribal perceptions of smallpox, around the early decades of the nineteenth century, the Kandhas for example identified it as a disease caused by Joogah Pennoo, the god of smallpox. Joogah Pennoo sowed smallpox just as men sowed seeds in the earth. We are told about the Kandhas deserting their villages when struck by smallpox. Those who remained made offerings of buffaloes, hogs, and sheep to appease the smallpox god. Kandhas of the neighbouring hamlets attempted to prevent Joogah Pennoo from reaching their village by planting thorns in the path that led to the affected village.[13] A part of their survival strategy made the Kandhas resort to the *meriah* (human) sacrifice, though the human component of this practice is contested by present-day anthropologists.[14] Although it is beyond the scope of this chapter to examine details associated with it, this sacrifice, amongst other things, sought to protect them from diseases.[15]

Similarly, the Kuttia Kandhas invented Dharma Pinnu – the smallpox goddess – to cope with the disease. Dharma Pinnu was seen as the source of smallpox and worshipped at all agricultural festivals. Interestingly, she was identified as an Oriya (Hindu) goddess living in the lap of luxury.[16] Ceremonies were performed in her honour just before sowing in the hill clearings. The invocations at her special ceremony were made in Oriya and the offerings were not the normal millet and rice beer, but milk, *ghee* (clarified butter), rice, and *mohwa* (liquor distilled from the mohwa tree).[17] That this reflected a part of a broader survival strategy becomes clear because tribals such as the Didayi also invented their goddess Mata, who represents a close parallel of the Dharma Pinnu of the Kandhas.[18]

When smallpox became virulent a little cart was made, on which a saffron-stained grain of rice representing every soul in the village was placed. After numerous offerings it was dragged with the necessary ceremonies to the boundary of the village. Through this the influence of the deity bringing smallpox was sought to be transferred across the village limits. Neighbouring villages followed this practice, moving the cart with the ceremonial accompaniments. After touring a whole set of villages the cart was abandoned in some lonely spot.[19] A similar trend has been observed in the Gujarat region by Hardiman, where the smallpox goddess was 'made' to enter a buffalo or goat and driven far away from the village. A more common practice was to entice her through offerings of food and sacrificial victims to quit the village. A large basket was filled with cooked rice and red powder. This was then taken to the border of the village, where it was buried. In some cases the basket passed from village to village till it reached the sea, where it was immersed.[20]

Another closely related method implied offering the smallpox goddess a sweet drink called *pana* (a ritualistic drink) at the junction of the roads leading away from the village. Through this the goddess, it was hoped, would leave the village without striking it with the dreaded disease. In fact, this latter method seems to have been adopted to keep out the goddesses of other diseases as well.[21]

What is also witnessed is that during the early 1860s the Kandhas of Subarnaghurry (Kandhamal) linked smallpox with the coming in of the Paikas – who had got both the disease and the 'sircar'. What followed included efforts to expel the Paikas. Additionally, there are references to some Kandhas of Pangoodah and Guddapoor being exploited by non-tribals, who inoculated them and charged fees that reduced many of them to poverty.[22]

For the Santals, the possibility of a smallpox epidemic saw the village elders getting together and agreeing to do something about it together. They declared themselves to be priests. After this, the headman got a priest who arranged for the necessary ingredients. On the next morning they assembled at the end of the village street with a brown female kid which was taken to the eastern boundary, and after she had grazed for a while she was taken around all the boundaries of the village. After this, she was decapitated and the remains were left there, which no one ate. If smallpox did not strike the village for a year then a goat and pigeons were sacrificed. In case smallpox did appear, then efforts were made to confine it to the person who had got the disease. An unmarried girl spun a cotton thread to which the medicine was tied to the patient, with chantings to Nag nagin and Kali mae. If the patient died it was supposed to be the handiwork of witches and recovery was attributed to an epidemic. Additionally, 'medicines' – which included black pepper, rice made from sun-dried paddy, etc. – were taken by everyone in the village. We also get references to several ways through which those having the disease could be made to feel comfortable while recovering. What is noticeable is the co-existence of a vegetarian diet with the animal/bird sacrifice, confining the disease to the patient, medicines that were distributed to everyone in the village with the hope that it worked as a prophylactic, and securing the village boundary to keep out the disease.[23]

Consequently, the dislocations affecting the tribal societies were reflected in some of the perceptions that we have sought to highlight. Nevertheless, the colonial order and the opposition to it was not mono-dimensional. Thus, the Kandhas associated the '*sircar*' – in metaphorical terms, colonialism – with smallpox, and this co-existed with knocking on the doors of the colonial establishment for help after trying out the non-tribal inoculators. Thus, what needs to be delineated here is that colonialism, which was associated with the new order, was feared, admired, revered, appeased, and also coaxed through a host of complex negotiations. Thus, one witnesses the awesome hold of colonial authority on tribal communities, co-existing with a subversive element when it comes to smallpox. Moreover, one cannot miss the association of smallpox with internal exploiters as well. However, to explain all these merely in terms of the intensity of the disease would be inadequate. It is of course worth speculating if the references to the village boundary and keeping out smallpox had anything to do with an awareness of human transmissibility. Nevertheless, what needs to be stressed is the fusion of a set of highly complex strands and that the 'resistance' to vaccination needs to be critiqued and problematized.

Smallpox and the colonial establishment

Smallpox vaccination was undoubtedly one of the most serious health interventions undertaken by the colonial administration in Orissa. Nevertheless, if we take the late eighteenth century as the starting point one gets a rather different picture. In fact, David Arnold refers to the favourable accounts (mostly by European doctors and surgeons) of variolation in eastern (and northern) India prior to 1800. Quoting extensively from the account of J. Z. Howell that he presented to the College of Physicians (London 1767), he cites the practice of this caste profession by a "particular tribe of Brahmins". They travelled from north India to Bengal and inoculated the patient's outer arm with 'variolous matter' collected from the previous year after making an incision with a metal instrument. This meant that that the patient got a mild attack of smallpox, which in fact produced a prophylactic effect. Arnold adds that this method of variolation was not carried out only by Brahmin inoculators, and that it protected about 60 percent of the population of Bengal and adjoining areas from smallpox. Besides, the British took up this practice in Calcutta and elsewhere in the late eighteenth century to protect themselves from smallpox. However, with the introduction of Edward Jenner's method of vaccination the colonialists tended to become sceptical and 'frankly contemptuous' of this rival practice.[24]

Thus, one can also see a meeting point between the Indian and European method of prevention of smallpox. This should make us careful about not over-emphasizing the dividing line often drawn between vaccination and inoculation. Alongside, resistance to vaccination needs to be also qualified and situated to accept a level of fluidities in the light of what we have discussed earlier – viz. the search for 'sircar vaccinators' by the Kandhas after being let down by non-tribal inoculators.[25]

Writing about smallpox, David Arnold also focuses on the conceptualization of the disease by the Indians and the Europeans. Thus, he delineates the importance of Sitala (the goddess of smallpox) and the fact that she was worshipped and propitiated – with smallpox being located as her divine presence rather than a disease. Moreover he points to the idea of a controlled and moderated form of the disease through variolation/inoculation, through live smallpox matter, to protect the individual against a subsequent attack.[26] He mentions various features such as the alienation of the vaccinators from the community, the unwillingness to expose women to vaccinators, and the failure rates of vaccination to explain the resistance to vaccination. However, his basic emphasis is on the 'raw secularity' that was associated with vaccination, that provoked resistance, wherein the goddess of smallpox did play a role.[27] Arnold also mentions the lack of preservation techniques which meant the low level of immunity for those who were vaccinated and the problems of creating a reliable vaccinating agency. As suggested, these problems were similar to Europe's own experience.[28] Arnold's position accommodates the improvement in preservation techniques with lymph being preserved in lanolin or glycerine that made vaccination more effective and acceptable.[29]

While focusing on the diversities associated with the process of vaccination itself, medical historians argue that in different parts of rural India it was really a form of inoculation. Thus, they refer to Reports from the localities in all the presidencies which often complained about the fact that local vaccinators had used humanized – and usually unattenuated – lymph when the preserved animal lymph transported from the district depots lost their potency. This unattenuated lymph could, and often did, have serious side effects, which, in turn, increased the opposition to a practice that was considered unreliable, especially when the unattenuated or inert lymph proved unable to provide resistance to smallpox after a painful operation. Given this, they emphasize the existence of a two-tiered system of vaccination, with an urban Vaccination Programme that was based on the current and tested technologies, and a rural vaccination scheme, where outdated and suspect technologies were often used.[30]

Mark Harrison is in fact quite critical about the manner in which historians have over-emphasized the cultural reasons for resistance to smallpox vaccination. He directs our attention to the grounds on which this was feared and resisted in Europe. Here he refers to the painful nature of the process, which was also accompanied by the possibilities of a secondary infection due to the vaccine being rendered ineffective, given the hot climatic conditions.[31]

Although we do not have statistical data for the Princely states during the nineteenth century, the point regarding the lymph losing its effectiveness is perhaps indicated by some of the sources which tell us about the hill tract of Ganjam, which form the basis of Table 4.1.[32] Thus, the gap between the number of people vaccinated and those in whose case it was reported to be 'successful' illustrates the problems associated with defective lymph supplies and the process of vaccination outside the urban centres. These points should be borne in mind while seeking to explain the opposition to vaccination. One should also reiterate a point already made earlier in this chapter about these years being marked by major rebellions, where the tribal people – including some in the Princely states – fought against colonialism and the new order that was being imposed on them.[33] This perhaps also explains the official position that was rather dismissive about the "apathy and indifference . . . [of the Kandhas] to submit to vaccination".[34] Consequently, the alternatives from the plains were tried, before knocking on the doors of the colonial administration for a '*sircar*' vaccinator, as has been already delineated.

Table 4.1 Statement showing the operation of vaccination in the hill tracts of Ganjam for the years 1882–1887

	1882–1883	*1883–1884*	*1886–1887*	*1887–1888*
Number vaccinated	5421	12571	4941	6066
Number successful	5134	12242	4764	5822

A virtually similar picture emerges when it comes to the tribal approach to the non-tribal people from the plains, some of whom were distinctly associated with their exploitation. This explains the anger against the Paikas, who were the favoured feudal retainers, settled in the hill tracts by the feudal chiefs. They were also hated because they were incorporated by and associated with the colonial agency. There is an observable link established in popular cosmology between the colonialist and the non-tribal exploiter when it came to identifying the outbreak of smallpox. Consequently, one needs to bear all these complexities in mind since many of the movements of the tribals over the nineteenth century were against both the internal and external exploiters, involving a wide range of tribal groups in western Orissa.

What perhaps also needs to be articulated is the approach to the problem of vaccination and the constraints it suffered from. One can cite here some details related to the colonial establishment's involvement to ameliorate the Kandhas who suffered due to the smallpox epidemic in the Ganjam tracts. In case of any such welfare schemes, the financial implications were carefully assessed. Thus, the concern about expenses occupied as important a position as the perception that this would be a 'boon' for the Kandhas.[35] At the same time, there were some in the medical establishment who did not exert themselves during the outbreak of smallpox and the sickness of some of the vaccinators, which sometimes constrained the operations. In other instances there was the problem of defective lymph supplies from Calcutta.[36] Consequently, given all these factors, one needs to be more open to questions related to the 'civilizing mission' and the very meaning of 'science' and 'progress' in the Adivasi world of colonial India.

The problems faced by this intervention are also visible from tracts in support of the vaccination drive, printed in Oriya at the Cuttack Mission Press. One such tract laments how only the *sahebs* (Westernized men) supported it, whereas the *murkhas* (uneducated) and the *agyani* (ignorant) people did not like vaccination. The author argued that it was the duty of all to first convince and explain to their domestic servants about the usefulness of vaccination. Moreover, when *tikadars* (vaccinators) visited villages, women hesitated to vaccinate children, which resulted in the large-scale death of children.[37] The system of vaccination implied a dependence on the zamindars since the colonial authorities felt that if persons of influence supported vaccination, it would find acceptability amongst the common people.[38] Alongside, the middle classes and the print-culture did to a certain extent legitimize the colonial interventions associated with smallpox.[39] Thus, the question from a maths textbook in Oriya has been cited at the very outset of this chapter as a clear example.

Some details related to Orissa and the Orissa Province (formed in 1936) here would perhaps help to illustrate the magnitude of the vaccination drive in the early twentieth century (see Table 4.2).[40]

Table 4.2 Number of vaccinations and re-vaccinations for the years 1906–1940

Year	Number of vaccinations	Number of re-vaccinations
1906–1907	165,967	43,498
1912–1913	387,190	215,438
1917–1918	526,410	330,938
1936–1937	603,006	–
1939–1940	706,275	–

This increase was not uncomplicated since we are told about the unpopularity of the vaccination fees "amongst all classes but especially among the poor" in north Orissa.[41] Although not grasped by the colonial officials, these sentiments seem to have been incorporated into the anti-imperialist struggle, if one goes by the decline in the number of people vaccinated in 1921 and 1929, years that converged with the mass Non-Cooperation Movement (1920–1922) and Civil Disobedience Movement (1929–1934) in Orissa.[42] Again, during the 1942 'Quit India' Movement a vaccinator was 'attacked' in parts of coastal Orissa.[43] Besides being seen as a symbol of the colonial state during this powerful, anti-colonial mass struggle, this act should be seen as responses to deeper problems posed by the colonial vaccination policy.

This picture would be incomplete unless the contestations against vaccination are delineated. As discussed, vaccination was much more than a substitution of one regulatory technology for another, especially since variolation involved an association with a religious act along with prevention, while vaccination was seen as a secular act that had an alien origin. Moreover, the latter's association with colonial state power reinforced this difference in perception.[44] The complication in case of defective lymph supplies as already discussed created the space for opposition. Besides, in some areas, such as the Princely state of Singhbhoom, the zamindars demanded 25 percent of the vaccination fees as they were opposed to the vaccination drive, since there were no fees charged.[45]

The restriction on inoculation was viewed in some quarters as an insult to Sitala.[46] The restrictions imposed by the colonial administration were violated as the inoculation process shifted from a public to a private affair. What is clearly observable is the virtual emergence of a subversive cult which aimed to continue with the indigenous system of inoculation. *Pujas* (religious ceremonies) with drums and cornets that accompanied them were no longer performed openly. Secret or hidden parts of the body came to be selected and the inoculation spot chosen changed from the forehead (viz. between the eyes) to the upper arm, knee, or the back of the hand. Another method of subversion was to reject government vaccinators on grounds of caste.[47] This does not appear to be convincing since we have already referred to Mastan Brahmins (who were cultivators and hence considered 'low' Brahmins) and Panas (untouchables) who were inoculators in the coastal tract and the Princely states, respectively.

In the twentieth century some shifts were visible. We have already mentioned the development of local governance and the associated Acts, the formation of the Orissa Province in 1936, and the installation of a popular Congress Ministry (1937–1939) in the chapter on leprosy. As has been suggested, the Government of India Act of 1919 was most significant since it devolved a number of administrative powers from the Centre to Provinces, by which the local self-governments were assigned the responsibilities of providing health services, including smallpox vaccination.[48] This implied the establishment of the new provincial vaccine institutes – the first of these was the King Institute of Guindy – a suburb in Madras city. In fact by 1932 there were lymph production centres in different provinces, including Bihar and Orissa (Namkum, near Ranchi), that produced vaccines, and by time of the Second World War the production and distribution reached its peak when the vaccine institutes had to meet the demands of the Allied army based in India.[49]

The Princely states

What is observable is that in the Princely states the Vaccination Programme made rapid strides.[50] Besides the fact that its "remarkable progress [was] under the supervision of the Political Agent",[51] it was the terror and coercion component that marked the triumph of colonial power/knowledge that frequently accompanied these drives. This situation seems to have continued right up to the early years of the twentieth century. Thus, in the Princely enclaves the vaccination drives often co-existed with the authoritarian practices and arbitrary taxes.[52] One can perhaps refer to Table 4.3 to illustrate this point:[53] The increasing number of vaccinations and re-vaccinations perhaps illustrate the manner in which this programme was pursued.

Table 4.3 Smallpox-related work done in the 'native' states under the supervision of the political agent (1906–1919)

Year	Total number of vaccinations	Total number of revaccinations
1	*2*	*3*
1906–1907	165,967	43,498
1907–1908	187,150	69,685
1908–1909	226,042	97,078
1909–1910	269,728	142,911
1910–1911	810,962	163,162
1911–1912	341,701	179,688
1912–1913	387,190	215,438
1913–1914	430,720	261,225
1914–1915	419,562	260,767
1915–1916	454,699	281,913
1916–1917	504,948	311,670
1917–1978	526,410	330,938
1918–1919	426,717	269,970

We would now explore some of the Princely states of Orissa to explore the way in which smallpox impacted them as well as the Vaccination Programme.

Gangpur

Although tribal society was tuned to patriarchal practices, the way smallpox polarized gender tensions in nineteenth-century Gangpur is rather striking. A reference from the early 1870s from Gangpur (a Princely state) provides evidence. When smallpox broke out in Kurumkel it was attributed to witches and the village headman sent four 'witch finders' who located four women. The headman sent a report to the Raja who sent an official (Gajendra Babu) to enquire, who, in turn, ordered all witches to restrain from any mischief and restore peace in the village. The matter seems to have attracted a lot of attention, since the Raja came over and camped at a nearby village.

Later, a small amount of hair was cut from the head of each of the four women who had been identified as witches and burnt. This was supposed to deprive the witches of their power. Then the four women were tied to posts and after being questioned were ritually tortured. One woman denied she was a witch and was beaten with a cane which split into two. After this she was beaten with the green stalk of a castor oil plant. After about half a dozen blows she confessed to being a witch and fainted on being released. Another woman had to go through the same ordeal and both of them died – one the next day and the other a few days later. Of the other two, one admitted that she was a witch and gave the names of the spirits responsible for the outbreak of smallpox, whereas the other denied any knowledge of witchcraft. Both were released with a warning and sacrifices were made to the *bhoots* (ghosts) named by the 'witch' after which '*saltanat* peace' returned to the village. What perhaps needs to be emphasized is that the Raja was fined Rs. 2,000/- and was awarded a year's Rigorous Imprisonment for his complicity in the matter, though he was not sent to the common jail but detained at Ranchi in Bihar.[54] This indicates the way the colonial establishment let off its collaborator (viz. the Raja of Gangpur) with a very mild punishment, although he was involved and sanctioned the torture of the women, two of whom were murdered.

The way tribal society consolidated its patriarchal position with the outbreak of smallpox illustrates its inner tensions and contradictions. The ritual torture of witches and symbolic cutting of their hair in order to deprive them of their power suggests a selective targeting of female identity. Besides, it seems that witchcraft enjoyed a fairly wide acceptance, if one bears in mind the role of the Gangpur Raja. Moreover, the measures taken against him by the colonial administration for the killing of the two 'witches' reveal a level of collaboration which was based on political constraints and considerations. These not only undermine the normally constructed image of the scientific and progress-based West, but also demonstrate the hollowness of the 'civilizing mission'.

Mayurbhanj

The early references from 1924–1925 suggest the high number of Adivasis who were treated in the medical establishments of the darbar (36,912). It had employed 24 licensed vaccinators and one female vaccinator, who together performed 27,461 vaccinations and went on tours.[55] Nevertheless, there was a 'virulent' epidemic of smallpox in 1926–1927.[56] This seems to have led to the appointment of some temporary paid vaccinators in 1929–1930. The Chief Medical Officer supervised the vaccination in the state. The darbar purchased 1,540 tubes of glycerinated lymph, spending Rs. 3,269.2.0. An amount of Rs. 6793.15.6 was spent on the Vaccination Programme.[57] At the beginning of 1935–1936 a smallpox epidemic broke out in 'some localities' and spread rapidly. There were 4,562 cases of people who were affected and there were 570 deaths. We are told about vaccination being offered free of cost, the tours, and the success of vaccination (viz. 94.96 percent) in the state. However, the critical reference to the public health system being "far from being satisfactory" seems to contradict all these steps. In fact, this needs to be located as a serious feature to explain the limitations of the darbar, along with the colonial health establishment, to improve the state of things.[58] In 1938–1939 the vaccinators toured the Sadr (224 days) and the interior areas such as Bamanaghati (250 days) and Pachipur (108 + 129 days during the year). The total number of vaccinations reached 89,547 (as against 89,430 during the previous year), with a 98.60 percent success in primary vaccinations and 98.47 percent success in re-vaccinations.[59] From 1941–1942 smallpox does not seem to have tormented the people of Mayurbhanj, and we get references to the vaccinators in the four subdivisions.[60]

Keonjhar

As for Keonjhar, it seems that an increasing number of the state's people visited the hospitals – which stood at 109,909 in 1933–1934 and 108,433 in 1934–1935 – which included different sections of the people. We are clearly told about smallpox vaccination being free and compulsory, and that 45,885 people were vaccinated (as against 43,064 the year before). The stress on tours by the medical establishment meant that the Medical Officer toured 23 days and the Chief Medical Officer toured 46 days during the year. There were 21,282 primary and 24,603 secondary vaccinations (as against 21,053 and 22,011, in 1933–1934, respectively). In fact, the total expenditure of the Vaccination Department stood at Rs. 3,767.14.0 (as against Rs. 3,602.9.0 the year before). However, 563 were affected by smallpox (which had increased from 363 in 1933–1934).[61]

By 1935–1936, there was one medical institution for 76,768 states people. The number of people vaccinated was 45,960, with a slight increase in the number of those affected by smallpox (viz. 716). The work done in Keonjhargarh and the outlying subdivisions of Champua and Anandapur were reported as 'fairly good' and they seem to be equipped with Infection Wards to keep patients of smallpox.[62] By 1937–1938 we are told about the 'growing popularity' of the medical institutions which were visited by 1,18,231 people and compared to the year 1933–1934, when 109,909 visited these. Besides, the number of people vaccinated stood at 48,326 – a slight decrease from the previous year (49,838), which was attributed to a vaccinator being ill. There was also saw a decline in the opposition to vaccination, and we are told about many "villagers [who] came up voluntarily to be vaccinated". There was no smallpox epidemic, but a few "sporadic cases" of smallpox from the three subdivisions, which affected 240 people (against 415 in the previous year).[63]

By 1938–1939, 28,768 males and 20,572 females were vaccinated, which assumes significance in the context of the colonial Vaccination Programme. As delineated, 1132 tubes of vaccine lymph and the tours related to the Programme meant an expenditure of Rs. 3925.2.0.[64] By 1939–1940 the Sadr Hospital had a refrigerator to preserve the sera and vaccine. Additionally, 1194 tubes of vaccine lymph were bought at Rs. 1496.12.0, and 29,404 males along with 19,460 females were vaccinated. The number of unsuccessful vaccinations was 5,544.[65] The Report of 1940–1941 attributed the appreciation of proper medical treatment and the popularity of the medical institutions in the 'interior' to the sub-assistant surgeon who toured the *hats* (viz. weekly markets). Smallpox seems to have died as an epidemic, with 1080 'sporadic' cases being reported from the three subdivisions.[66] Thus, by 1941–1942 smallpox seems to have lost the label of an epidemic – even in the interiors of the state, with 847 cases being reported.[67]

Kalahandi

With ten dispensaries, two of which were located in the Headquarters (Bhawanipatana) and eight in the interiors, including five in the zamindaris, Kalahandi attended to 1,77,583 patients in 1933–1934 (as against 1,42,830 patients in 1932–1933). This was attributed to "the growing popularity" of the health system which brought in "patients from [the] bordering British District, other States and Agency tracts for treatment" to Bhawanipatana. We are told about a smallpox epidemic that could be checked due to vaccination. Vaccination was free and compulsory. There were 17 male and three female full-time vaccinators, who were supervised by the Chief Medical Officer. The total number of vaccinations stood at 63,216 (which was 58,859 in the previous year). The state got its lymph supplies from the Depot at Namkum, for which Rs. 730 was spent (as against Rs. 1081.10.0 in the previous year).[68] The *Report for 1940–41* provides details of the expenditure on the dispensaries in the five zamindaries.[69]

The *Report of 1941–42* mentions that there were 43,223 vaccinations (as against 41,280 in the previous year). The state saw 24,924 primary vaccinations out of which 24,013 were successful and 587 were unsuccessful. Besides, 18,299 were revaccinated; out of this 17,179 were successful and 690 were unsuccessful and no information was available for 430.[70] The *Report for 1945–46* referred to smallpox as a disease plaguing the state. Out of 23,931 vaccinations 22,628 were successful and 884 were unsuccessful and there was no information for 409. As delineated, after a successful vaccination, a revaccination was performed after an interval of seven years. The total number of re-vaccinations stood at 19,994 out of which 18,264 were successful and 1089 unsuccessful and there was no information for 614.[71]

Next we take up some of the Princely states that saw powerful prajamandal (viz. state people's) movements. The paucity of sources prior to the period that is examined was the result of these despotic enclaves not keeping any records in a systematic manner prior to the 1930s. We should also bear in mind that the praja-mandal movement created an indirect pressure on the darbars since their counter-offensives sought to divide the prajamandals through the creation of parallel bodies that they could control. This meant that some concessions in the form of health and education had to be in turn factored in. These were also necessary to reinforce the links between the darbars with the colonial government, and *vice versa*, after the 1937–1938 phase and which lasted till the 1942 Movement – which was undoubt-edly the most powerful mass movement witnessed by the colonial government and some of the darbars.[72]

Nilgiri

In 1940–1941, Nilgiri had two male and one female vaccinator, which saw an increase during the smallpox season (viz. October to March), when there were four male and two female vaccinators. The number of those vaccinated included 15,155; out of this 13,520 were successful. Vaccine lymph worth Rs. 455.2.0 was bought from the Government Vaccine Depot at Namkum.[73] As reported, in 1941–1942, 17,423 people were vaccinated out which 15,887 were successful.[74] And, with one head vaccinator and three permanent vaccinators (one male and two female) and three temporary vaccinators in 1942–1943, the number of the vac-cinated stood at 17,021 out of which 15,283 were successful.[75] These steps seem to be connected to the absence of any smallpox epidemic, though 97 people got smallpox and 20 of them died in 1943–1944,[76] 23 people died in 1944–1945, and 37 lives were lost in 1945–1946 due to smallpox.[77]

Dhenkanal

As for Dhenkanal, we are told about the absence of any epidemic in 1932–1933. There were four charitable dispensaries along with one hospital each at the Head-quarters, and in the interior at Murhi, Bhuban, and Bhaupur. The medical staff toured fairs and *hatas* and distributed medicines. The total number of patients who were attended to stood at 80,473, which included 360 indoor patients. The expen-diture of the Medical Department stood at Rs. 18,445.4.8. Along with vaccination tours, 22,264 were vaccinated and there were 8595 primary and 13,669 cases of re-vaccination; besides, the total number of women vaccinated stood at 8,439.[78] *The Report of 1933–34* refers to the medical establishment's efforts to 'train' as many 'local people' as possible to work for it. There were 19 licensed vaccina-tors who had vaccinated 23,452 people, out of which 9,309 were women.[79] The *Report of 1942–43* refers to two Pana (Untouchable caste) vaccinators along with two female and 20 temporary, licensed vaccinators. As reported, "vaccination was practically compulsory". There was a smallpox epidemic in the mofussils (village tracts) and 114 people lost their lives. The state people paid "Rs.0.1.6 for each suc-cessful case" of vaccination in the working season and during "the non-working season" it "was free of cost".[80] *The Report for 1944–45* referred to the Pana vacci-nators continuing with vaccination, with one of them working during the 'working season' – viz. 15 October to 15 March. The total number of primary vaccination was 8,094 and there were 20,952 re-vaccinations. The total expenditure incurred stood at Rs. 3,975, which included the cost of lymph – Rs. 2,425. There was no epidemic and the number of deaths from smallpox stood at 21.[81]

Conclusion

This chapter explored the processes and the complexities generated by the inter-actions between colonialism, the Adivasi and the non-tribal population, and the bearing they had on smallpox, focusing on some of the Princely states. Certain points clearly emerge from our discussion. It needs to be reiterated that instead of posing inoculation and vaccination as binaries, one perhaps needs to see major meeting points between them, especially in the nineteenth century. As observed, the responses of the Adivasis and the people in the margins to the colonial vac-cination policy over the nineteenth century reflected deeper problems posed by colonialism and its internal collaborators.

We have also noted the logic of Hinduization and conversion of the Adivasis and the latter's efforts to get incorporated within the Brahminical order, with the evolution of smallpox goddesses amongst the tribal communities. The fact that the world of the Adivasis was rather vulnerable when it comes to smallpox prevention needs to be noted.

The role of the Outcastes and Untouchables – especially those like the Haliya Brahmins or the Panas – and their expertise insofar as inoculation is concerned has been highlighted. We see the examples of the Low/Outcastes possibly gaining the status of Low/Haliya Brahmins and Panas in some of the Princely states as acceptable inoculators. Thus, the reference to Pana inoculators being trained and recruited as vaccinators by the medical establishments of some of the Princely states suggests their incorporation by the darbars and the colonial establishment. This questions the often-cited rigid hold of the order of caste and illustrates the existence of fluidities that implied a level of not only accommodation, but also the acceptance of the demonized and humiliated 'Others' while facing a dreaded disease. Consequently, one needs to be cautious about the resistance to vaccination on grounds of caste. And while discussing this point, one needs to add that perhaps the idea of having women vaccinators did play a role in the acceptance of the Vac-cination Programme by sections of women in the Princely states.

We have noted the terror struck by the colonial inroads in the hills of Orissa till the 1860s that made the Adivasis suspicious and wary of the Vaccination Pro-gramme. Besides this, the lack of preservation techniques made the vaccines inef-fective and naturally caused anxieties when smallpox affected a person after a painful process associated with vaccination. In fact the problems and insecurities were related to the workings of the vaccination policy, which meant – outside the urban environment – defective lymph supplies and the problem of getting smallpox, even after the painful process of vaccination. These problems did get somewhat altered with the improvement of preservation techniques and the open-ing of a Vaccine Depot at Namkum (as has been already mentioned), and some states procuring refrigerators to store the vaccines. Nevertheless, the references to 'successful'/'unsuccessful' vaccinations in some Reports in the early 1940s illustrate how the smallpox Vaccination Programme suffered serious setbacks.

This chapter also highlighted how health issues can become part of discriminatory practices directed at women, who are located as the 'Other'. The way smallpox was identified with witches and led to the torture and the murder of two women indicates this, in the context of tribal society. That non-tribal Oriya (Hindu) society located the male child as hierarchically superior is evidenced in the way higher inoculation fees were paid for boys. This perhaps illustrates how patriarchy subsumes social differences and targets women, irrespective of whether they are tribals or non-tribals.

At the outset we have referred to the efforts of some Adivasis such as the Kandhas to try out inoculation and then look for *sircar* (government) vaccinators. We can end by referring to the shifts and changes in the political and social life of the people that altered the shape and in turn conditioned the way the colonial Vaccination Programme was re-shaped. However, to attribute its success to improved technology alone, or see it as a success of the 'civilizing mission' would mean seeing the tip of the proverbial iceberg. After all, Sitala and Dharma Pinnu did have a long life – longer than what had been perhaps anticipated – if one goes by the fact that the WHO declared the successful eradication of smallpox in India only in 1980.

Notes

1 Radhanath Ray, *Ardhaprasnabali Part 1*, Balasore 1878, Vernacular Tracts, India Office Collection, British Library (London), 19; translation mine.
2 Angela K.C. Leung, '"Variation" and Vaccination in Late Imperial China, Ca. 1570–1911', in Stanley A. Plotkin (ed.), *History of Vaccine Development*, New York: Springer, 2011, 5; 8 (5–12).
3 Luise White, *Speaking With Vampires: Rumor and History in Colonial Africa*, Berkeley: University of California Press, 2000, 102.
4 Jonathan B. Tucker, *Scourge: The Once and Future Threat of Smallpox*, New York: Grove Press, 2002, 18.
5 Harve Bazim, *Vaccination: A History – From Lady Montagu to Genetic Engineering*, Montrouge: John Libbey Eurotext, 2011, 29–30; 33–6.
6 We can refer here to David Arnold (ed.), *Imperial Medicine and Indigenous Societies*, New Delhi: Oxford University Press, 1989; and his *Colonising the Body: State Medicine and Epidemic Disease in Nineteenth Century India*, Berkeley: University of California Press, 1993.
7 Biswamoy Pati, 'Siting the Body: Perspectives on Health and Medicine in Colonial Orissa', in Biswamoy Pati, *Situating Social History: Orissa, 1800–1997*, Hyderabad: Orient Longman, 2001, 1–25; Niels Brimnes, 'Variolation, Vaccination and Popular Resistance in Early Colonial South India', *Medical History*, 48(2), 2004, 199–228; Christiana Bastos, 'Borrowing, Adapting, and Learning the Practices of Smallpox: Notes From Colonial Goa', *Bulletin of the History of Medicine*, 83(1), 2009, 140–63.
8 K.N. Panikkar, 'Indigenous Medicine and Cultural Hegemony' in his *Culture, Ideology, Hegemony: Intellectuals and Social Consciousness in Colonial India*, New Delhi: Tulika, 1995, 145–75; Niels Brimnes, 'Variolation, Vaccination and Popular Resistance in Early Colonial South India', *Medical History*, 48(2), 2004, 199–228; and 'The Sympathising Heart and the Healing Hand: Smallpox Prevention and Medical Benevolence

in Early Colonial South India', in Harald Fischer-Tine and Michael Mann (eds.), *Colonialism as Civilising Mission: Cultural Ideology in British India*, London: Anthem, 2004, 191–204; Perundevi Srinivasan, 'Constructing Goddess Worship', in Sree Padma (ed.), *Inventing and Reinventing the Goddess: Contemporary Iterations of Hindu Deities on the Move*, Maryland: Lexington Books, 2014, 68–81 (63–88).

9   Sanjoy Bhattacharya, 'Re-devising Jennerian Vaccines? European Technologies, Indian Innovation and the Control of Smallpox in South Asia, 1850–1950', in Biswamoy Pati and Mark Harrison (eds.), *Health, Medicine and Empire: Perspectives on Colonial India*, New Delhi: Orient Longman, 2001, 217–69.

10   Arnold, *Colonising the Body*, correctly speaks of a method that should not compartmentalize the Western and the Indian system but accept interactions, 291. However, as we shall see, this itself simplifies things since his method does not seem to recognize the complexities and pluralities, in the context of the tribal communities. The method of K.N. Panikkar, 'Indigenous Medicine and Cultural Hegemony', recognizes this dimension.

11   This has remarkable continuities even amongst present-day scholars P.K. Nayak and Anil Mahajan (eds.), *Human Encounter With Drought*, New Delhi: Reliance Publishing House, 1991, 119, who, for example refer to the "villagers" in the Kalahandi region being "totally in darkness in regard to modern concept of health and disease".

12   Very few scholars seem to view things holistically – disease, colonial wars directed against the Adivasis, and the shifts and changes that these reinforced; one can refer to exceptions here such as Sumit Guha, 'Forest Politics and Agrarian Empires: The Khandesh Bhills, c.1700–1850', *Indian Economic and Social History Review*, 33(2), 1996, 345–59 and David Arnold, 'Disease, Resistance and India's Ecological Frontier, 1770–1947', in Biswamoy Pati (ed.), *Issues in Modern Indian History: For Sumit Sarkar*, Bombay: Popular Prakashan, 2000, 1–22.

13   S.C. MacPherson, *Report Upon the Khonds of the Districts of Ganjam and Cuttack*, Calcutta: Military Orphan Press, 1842, 69.

14   See G. Pfeffer, 'Kondh Classification and Mythology in Macpherson's "Account"', in M. Brandtner and S.K. Panda (eds.), *Interrogating History: For Hermann Kulke*, New Delhi: Manohar, 2006, 347–64.

15   European MSS D/1112, Extract from dispatch, dated 19 February, 1837 . . . from Henry Ricketts, Commissioner Cuttack, to the Government of India; India Office Library (hereafter IOL) London. One might add here that the *meriah* sacrifice was also supposed to ensure good crops and prevent accidents.

16   Dharma Pinnu should not be in any way mistaken with Laxmi – the Hindu goddess of prosperity and wealth. Note: the difference in spelling between Pennoo (in case of Joogah Pennoo) and Pinnu is because I have retained the way they are referred to in the sources.

17   N.A. Watts, *The Half Clad Tribes of Eastern India*, Bombay: Orient Longman, 1970, 65.

18   Uma Guha, M.K.A Siddiqui and P.R.G. Mathur, *The Didayi: A Forgotten Tribe of Orissa*, New Delhi: Anthropological Survey of India, 1968, 186.

19   Nrusinha Charan Behuria, *Final Report on the Major Settlement Operations in Koraput District 1938–64*, Cuttack: Orissa Government Press, 1966, 30.

20   David Hardiman, *The Coming of the Devi: Adivasi Assertion in Western India*, New Delhi: Oxford University Press, 1987, 25–6.

21   Kunja Bihari Das and L.K. Mahapatra, *Folklore of Orissa*, New Delhi: National Book Trust, 1979, 100; the reference to the other disease include chickenpox, cholera, measles and the plague epidemic.

22   Home Dep.(Public Branch), nos. 60–61 (A), 24 January, 1861, National Archives of India, New Delhi; hereafter NAI.

23   P.O. Bodding, *Studies in Santal Medicine and Connected Folklore, Parts I, II and III*, Kolkata: The Asiatic Society, 2011 (originally published in 1925–40), 276–80.

24 David Arnold, *The New Cambridge History of India: III. 5 Science, Technology and Medicine in Colonial India*, Cambridge: Cambridge University Press, 2000, 72–3.

25 Home Dep. (Public Branch), nos. 60–61 (A), 24 January, 1861, NAI.

26 David Arnold, *Colonising the Body*, 120; 126. Whereas inoculation, operated with the method of crust collection and a process that required special skill and was a caste profession, including in colonial Orissa, vaccination was associated with the colonial health establishment and a technological process, which prepared the vaccine using animal lymph.

27 Arnold, *Colonising the Body*, 143.

28 *Ibid.*, 156.

29 David Arnold, *The New Cambridge History of India: Science, Technology and Medicine in Colonial India*, Cambridge: Cambridge University Press, 2000, 75.

30 Sanjoy Bhattacharya, 'Re-devising Jannerian Vaccines? European Technologies, Indian Innovation and the Control of Smallpox in South Asia, 1850–1950', *Social Scientist*, 28(306–307), 1998, 27–66.

31 Mark Harrison, *Disease and the Modern World: 1500 to the Present*, Cambridge: Polity Press, 2014, 96.

32 Based on Ganjam District Records, Orissa State Archives (hereafter OSA), Bhubaneshwar, Accession nos. 1292G and 1953G.

33 These features perhaps reached their peak during the 1857 Rebellion; for details see, Biswamoy Pati, 'Beyond Colonial Mapping: Common People, Fuzzy Boundaries and the Rebellion of 1857', in Biswamoy Pati (ed.), *The Great Rebellion of 1857: Exploring Transgressions, Contests and Diversities*, Oxford: Routledge, 2010, 46–62.

34 This reference is based on an official note of the Inspector of Vaccination and Deputy Sanitary Commissioner, Ganjam, February 1880; cited in Acc. no. 1871, Ganjam District Records (OSA);

35 Home Dep. (Public Branch), nos. 60–61 (A) 24 Jan.1861, NAI; thus, as calculated by the colonial administration, engaging three vaccinators for the Kandhas of the hill tracts of Orissa would mean an expenditure of Rs. 400/- annually (viz. Rs.10/- per month as their salary + other expenditure). While discussing the hurdles met by the vaccination policy Arnold, *Colonising the Body* also mentions the reluctance of the colonial state to shoulder the financial burden of mass vaccination; 121.

36 Home Dep.(Sanitary Branch), nos. 7–10, November1881, Home Dep.(Medical Branch), nos. 68–71 Part (A)January1880 – 'Report on Vaccination – Bengal 1878–79'; NAI.

37 John Shortt, *Tika Deba Bisae Bidhan* (Oriya: A Popular Treatise on Vaccination in Oriya), Cuttack: Orissa Mission Press, 1867, 3; 9; Vernacular Tracts, India Office Collection, British Library (London), translation mine.

38 Home Dep.(Sanitary Branch), nos.7–10, Nov.1881, NAI.

39 Thus Arnold, *Colonising the Body*, 157, suggests that by the 1880s Indian middle classes began to support the vaccination policy.

40 Based on S.N. Tiwari, *Annual Statistical Returns and Short Notes on Vaccination in Bihar and Orissa for the Year 1918–19*, Patna: Superintendent of Government Printing, 1919, 3; G. Verghese, *Annual Public Health Report of the Province of Orissa for the Year 1936 the Vaccination Report for the Year1936–37*, Cuttack: Orissa Government Press, 1938, 19; G. Verghese, *Annual Public Health Report of the Province of Orissa for the Year1939 and the Annual Vaccination Report for the Year 1939–40*, Cuttack: Orissa Government Press, 1941, 33.

41 G. Verghese, *Annual Public Health Report*, 36.

42 W.C. Ross, *Annual Sanitary Report of the Province of Bihar and Orissa for the Year 1921*, Patna: Superintendent of Government Printing, 1922, 3, and J.A.S. Phillips, *Annual Public Health Report of the Province of Bihar and Orissa for the Year 1928 and the Annual Vaccination Report for the Year 1928–29*, Patna: Superintendent of Government Printing, 1923, do refer to the decline in the number of people vaccinated.

Needless to say 1929–1931 were years of acute economic pressures, with the colonial economy reeling under the throes of the 'Great Depression'.

43 Biswamoy Pati, *Resisting Domination: Peasants, Tribals and the National Movement in Orissa, 1920–50*, New Delhi: Manohar, 1993, 164.

44 Arnold, *Colonising the Body*, 120.

45 Home Dep.(Medical Branch), nos. 68–71 Part (A)January1880 – 'Report on Vaccination – Bengal 1878–79'; NAI. Note: Singhbhoom was a princely state of Orissa that merged with Bihar after Independence.

46 In fact, Marglin, 'Smallpox in Two Systems', 139 echoes this sentiment. Hardiman, *The Coming of the Devi*, 24; 52–4 refers to the feeling amongst the village folk of Gujarat that government methods of restricting her progress would enrage Sitala. This got polarised with the Devi spreading the message of the 'mahatma' (M.K. Gandhi), getting associated with social reform and emerging as the vehicle of protest against the Parsi exploiters by 1921–1922. However, this trend was not visible in Orissa.

47 Home Dep.(Medical Branch), nos. 68–71 Part (A) Jan.1880 NAI; interestingly, the reference is to people asking for a Brahmin vaccinator, but refusing his services after he joined.

48 Chandrakant Lahariya, 'A Brief History of Vaccines & Vaccination in India', *Indian Journal of Medical Research*, 139(4), 2014, 491–511; thus, the health service delivery sector being a 'State subject' in India had its origin in this Act.

49 Sanjoy Bhattacharya, Mark Harrison and Michael Worboys, *Fractured Sites: Smallpox, Public Health and Vaccination Policy in British India, 1800–1947*, Hyderabad: Orient Longman, 2005, 191–2.

50 L.E.B. Cobden Ramsay, *Bengal Gazetteers: Feudatory States of Orissa*, Calcutta, 1910, reprinted Calcutta: Firma K.L.M., 1982, 70.

51 W.C. Ross, *Annual Sanitary Report 1916*, Patna: Superintendent Government Printing, 1917, 32.

52 This enthusiasm for smallpox vaccination was true for many of the princely states, especially in the context of the nineteenth century when they were hardly concerned about the health of the people in the states. The case of the zamindars of Singhbhoom has been already cited. Besides, we get references to 'invisible' charges related to Nilgiri, which included 'medical' charges; for details, H.K. Mahtab, Balvantray Mehta and Lalmohan Patnaik, *Report of the Enquiry Committee: Orissa States*, Cuttack: Orissa Mission Press, 1939, 11–12.

53 Based on S.N. Tiwari, *Annual Statistical Returns and Short Notes on Vaccination in Bihar and Orissa for the Year 1918–19*, Patna: Superintendent Government Printing, 1919, 3.

54 C.L. Philips, 'Confidential History of Gangpur State' (up to 1927), Crown Representative Papers, R/2 306/121, undated, IOL, London; Indrabilas Mukherji, *Final Report on the Land Revenue Settlement of the Gangpur State, 1929–1936*, Berhampur: Indian Law Publication Press, 1938, 5, contains a brief reference to this incident.

55 *Report on the Administration of Mayurbhanj, 1924–25*, Baripada: State Press Mayurbhanj, 1925, 70; 73; 75.

56 Mohammed Laeequddin, *Census of Mayurbhanj State, 1931, Vol. I*, Calcutta: Calendonian Printing Company, 1937, 11.

57 *Report on the Administration of Mayurbhanj, 1929–30*, Baripada: State Press Mayurbhanj, 1930, 82.

58 *Report on the Administration of Mayurbhanj, 1935–36*, Baripada: State Press Mayurbhanj, 1939, 85–7.

59 *Report on the Administration of Mayurbhanj, 1938–39*, Baripada: State Press Mayurbhanj; Calcutta: Bani Press, 1941, 73–4.

60 *Report on the Administration of Mayurbhanj, 1941–42*, Baripada: State Press Mayurbhanj, 1944, 99.

61 *Review and Report of the Administration of the Keonjhar State for 1934–35*, Lucknow: The Pioneer Press, 1936, 36–9.

62 *Review and Report of the Administration of the Keonjhar State for 1935–36*, Keonjhargarh: State Press, 1936, 45–6.

63 *Annual Report on the Administration of the Keonjhar State for 1937–38*, Keonjhargarh: State Press, 1939, 42; 44–5.

64 *Annual Report on the Administration of the Keonjhar State for 1938–39*, Keonjhargarh: State Press, 1940, 44.

65 *Annual Report on the Administration of the Keonjhar State for 1939–40*, Keonjhargarh: State Press, 1942, 47; 48.

66 *Annual Report on the Administration of the Keonjhar State for 1940–41*, Keonjhargarh: State Press, 1942, 39; 43.

67 *Annual Report on the Administration of the Keonjhar State for 1941–42*, Keonjhargarh: State Press, 1943, 51.

68 *Report on the Administration of Kalahandi for the Year 1933–34*, Kalahandi State Press: Place and Year of Publication not mentioned, 48; 50; 52.

69 *Report on the Administration of Kalahandi for the Year 1940–41*, Cuttack: Saraswati Press, 1941, 40.

70 *Report on the Administration of Kalahandi for the Year 1941–42*, Bhawanipatana: Kalahandi State Press, 1943, 55.

71 *Report on the Administration of Kalahandi for the Year 1945–46*, Bhawanipatana: Kalahandi State Press, Year of Publication not mentioned, 49.

72 For details Pati, *Resisting Domination*, 86–205.

73 *Administration Report of the Nilgiri State Eastern States Agency the Year 1940–41*, Balasore: Town Press, 1941, 10.

74 *Administration Report of the Nilgiri State ESA for the Year 1941–42*, Balasore: Town Press, 1942, 15.

75 *Administration Report of the Nilgiri State ESA for the Year 1942–43*, Balasore: Town Press, 1944, 19.

76 *Administration Report of the Nilgiri State ESA for Year 1943–44*, Balasore: Town Press, 1944, 28–9.

77 *Administration Report of the Nilgiri State ESA for Year 1944–45*, Nilgiri: Nilgiri Darbar, no date of publication mentioned, 53; *Administration Report of the Nilgiri State ESA for Year 1945–46*, Balasore: Town Press, no date of publication mentioned, 52.

78 *The Report on the Administration of the Dhenkanal State for the Year 1932–33*, Dhenkanal: State Jail Press, 1933, 17–19.

79 *Report on the Administration of the Dhenkanal State for the Year 1933–34*, Dhenkanal: Sankar Press, Sadar Jail, 1934, 35–6.

80 *The Report on the General Administration of the Dhenkanal State for the Year 1942–43*, Dhenkanal: Sankar Press Sadar Jail, 1943, 28.

81 *Dhenkanal State Administrative Report for 1944–45*, Dhenkanal: Sankar Press, Sadar Jail, 1945, 42.

Section 3

Travancore and Orissa

Waltraud Ernst

5 Medical developments and Western psychiatry in Travancore and Orissa

Introduction

Following his visit to South Asia in 1937/8, the eminent British psychiatrist, Edward Mapother, commented on the conditions prevalent in a number of mental hospitals in Ceylon (Sri Lanka), British India and the Indian Princely states. He considered Mysore as "well ahead of any part of British India as regards the prosperity of its people" and its mental institution as "exceptional".[1] Travancore he described as "one of the most progressive states in India", with the lowest proportion of illiteracy in the whole of South Asia.[2] Conversely, he referred to Udaipur (Mewar) as "a picturesque survival of primitive conditions",[3] suggesting that it "might be interesting as a place for any scientific investigation which required primitive conditions for comparison".[4] Mapother's attention focused on the efficient organization of medical services and scientific psychiatric research, which were seen by him to be present in their most developed form in the United States, and in Continental European countries such as Germany, and, of course, in his own institution in England, the Maudsley Mental Hospital. To him states such as Mewar, which he thought were "almost unchanged by the advent of Europeans", constituted the antithesis to socially and medically advanced Mysore and Travancore.[5] Reputedly 'backward' Indian states without any institutional provision for the mentally ill, such as those in the non-British areas of Orissa, did not figure at all in his appraisal.

Mapother's reflections lacked the authority of an official government report and were based on cursory observations, skewed judgements, and a restricted source base. Nevertheless, his unpublished manuscript on a select number of mental institutions in India documents the diversity of conditions prevalent in different areas of the Subcontinent.[6] Even in provinces directly ruled by the British, 'colonial psychiatry' was not one thing but many, and conditions and treatments in the nineteen institutions maintained by the colonial power in the 1930s varied considerably. Conditions in mental hospitals in some of the Indian Princely states were considered comparable, if not superior, to those prevalent in particular British-run mental hospitals. Others were seen as backward, even primitive, as were the states in which they were located.

Mapother was known for his strong, partisan views and outspokenness.[7] Nonetheless, his accounts highlight issues that are central to some of the questions explored in this chapter. First, how did the provisions made for the mentally ill in Indian Princely states compare to those available in British India? Second, how did the different kinds of psychiatric services available in Indian-ruled India compare to each other? It will be shown that neither British nor Princely India's mental health provision was consistently progressive or backward. Both possessed their share of "enlightened" or "modern" facilities and of commendably patient-friendly services and doctors, as well as examples of "wretched provision" and "ignorance and indifference" amongst medical men.[8] It will be argued that 'colonial psychiatry' and 'psychiatry in Princely India' are umbrella terms. Like 'British psychiatry' or 'German psychiatry' or even 'Western psychiatry', they privilege national provenance and ideological context. However, they do not articulate the multifaceted realities of local politics, ideas, ideologies, and practices, or the plurality of medical agency. A comprehensive assessment of these issues requires analysis of the wider medical context within which psychiatric provision developed at particular localities, as well as an examination of the economic and socio-political affairs that framed them.

A 'modern' and 'ideal' Indian state: Travancore

Colonialism thrived on ideological bifurcations that juxtaposed the British rulers' enlightened qualities with the ostensibly inferior and backward characteristics of indigenous despots and colonized peoples. However, there were exceptions. Much patronizing praise was bestowed on areas ruled by Princes who were open to collaboration with the British or bullied through subsidiary alliances into the adoption of certain features of Western-style modernity. The major states given the title 'progressive' by the British were Baroda, Mysore, Travancore, and Cochin. Progress meant, as Ramusack notes, "administrative modernisation with some introduction of representative institutions", even if most princes remained autocrats who allowed little political participation.[9] Adjustments in the spheres of trade, industry, and agriculture were considered no less important. Travancore constituted a desirable area for traders and merchants, being rich in pepper, cardamom, and wood products.[10] To the delight of colonial investors it also lent itself to the cultivation of rubber, tea, and coffee. However, the existing state monopoly on agricultural products was detrimental to British interests. It came to an end when British annexation of the state was threatened and averted only by a drastic change in state policy by Dewan Madava Raw (Rao) (1828–1891): foreign trade and investment was to be encouraged. Madava Rao, who administered Travancore from 1857 to 1872 under Uthram and then Ayilyam Thirunal's rule, had been educated in British India, at Madras Government High School (later Presidency College). As Griffith, author of *India's Princes*, put it in 1894, he "proved himself to be a statesman and organiser of the greatest ability".[11] He devised policies that pleased the British:

> He quickly abolished trade monopolies, did away with vexatious taxes and restrictions which hampered the commercial success of the country, and by

this so stimulated industry that under his wise rule European coffee and tea cultivators were induced to settle in the state and to buy land. Public buildings sprang up everywhere, roads were laid out, and bridges and canals built, and the state treasury became full.[12]

Griffith added, virtually as an afterthought that reads like an attempt to ennoble the Dewan's trade-focused concerns: "and the grievances of the poor were redressed".[13] In fact, Travancore gained recognition for its remarkable expansion of social welfare measures between the 1860s and 1940s. This, together with Christian missionary endeavours, is seen by some academics as the basis on which post-colonial Kerala could gain its reputation as an "exceptionally" developed region when the state of Travancore became part of the new Indian state in 1949 alongside Princely Kochin.[14] Usually Travancore's late nineteenth- and early twentieth-century modernization along Western lines has been attributed to its monarchy's enlightened attitude. The records are full of praise by eminent British officials to that effect. For example, Eton, Sandhurst, and Addiscombe-educated Commander-in-Chief Lord Frederick Roberts' view of the learned and English-educated Maharaja Visakham Thirunal (1837–1885) was that,

> The late Maharajah was an unusually enlightened Native. He spoke and wrote English fluently; his appearance was distinguished and his manners those of a well-bred courteous English gentleman of the old school. His speech on proposing the Queen's health was a model of fine feeling and fine expression.[15]

In a sweeping gesture of disparagement of Indians in general, Roberts (who had served during the Indian Rebellion, the Second Boer War, and in Abyssinia and Afghanistan) elevated Thirunal on account of his exhibition of features of Englishness.[16] In a similar vein, Sir M.E. Grant Duff, Governor of Madras from 1881–1886, typecast the Maharaja, also known as Rama Varma the Learned, as "a typical example of the influence of English thought upon the South Indian mind".[17] A couple of decades earlier, Lord Francis Napier (Governor of Madras from 1866–1872), when visiting Travancore's capital Trivandrum (Thiruvananthapuram), commended the elder brother preceding Rama Varma from 1860–1880, Maharaja Ayilyam Thirunal (1832–1880), during his banquet speech in February 1868:

> You have all been witnesses of the examples of a humane and enlightened administration of which the capital is the scene. I will only notice a peculiar feature in His Highness' course which is very rare in the history of reforming Princes. The Maharajah has held a judicious and prudent middle way, avoiding all extremes; conservative by temperament, liberal by intelligence, he preserves the confidence of his own people, while he satisfies abroad the discriminating expectation of a progressive age.[18]

The profits that Western planters and foreign capital were able to realize were overlooked in smarmy toasts to persons whose continued rule depended on subservience to British colonial authorities. Furthermore, land tenure reforms and the expansion of education and healthcare had been vitally fuelled by the rulers' ambition to avoid annexation by the British. The reforms also strengthened the perceived legitimacy of the monarchy in the eyes of those who were becoming increasingly attuned to Western understandings of governance; not least on account of missionary initiatives against slavery and caste discrimination. As Desai suggests in regard to the land reforms in 1865, rulers' "deep structural reforms cannot be abstracted from their peculiarly dependent position upon the British".[19]

Travancore's dependence on British goodwill had begun with a treaty of subsidiary alliance with the East India Company in 1795 when threatened with invasion by Mysore's Tipu Sultan. Travancore was forced to accept a British resident in 1800.[20] By quelling an upper-caste mutiny (Nair or Nayar revolt) against the Princely ruler in 1804, the British established paramountcy over Travancore state.[21] Subsequently, in 1810, Maharani Lakshmi Bayi (1791–1815), Travancore's then queen, declared somewhat fawningly yet with an acute sense for *realpolitik* that the East India Company's "bosom had been an asylum for the protection of an infant like Travancore", putting herself gratefully under its "guidance and support".[22] As Fisher has shown, indirect rule via the British resident, John Munro, was highly interventionist, with policies modelled on those in British India, in particular neighbouring Madras presidency.[23] The reforms he suggested between 1811 and 1819 included reorganization of the police, judicial, and revenue systems, abolition of slavery in some parts of the country, and creation of the Vaccination Department.[24] Munro was also on good terms with the local missionaries, leading his fellow Scot Charles Grant, evangelical reformer and director of the East India Company, to support his appointment as honorary life-governor of the Church Missionary Society on his return to England in 1819.[25] In his praise, the *Missionary Register* declared that

> He [John Munro] has manifested the wisdom and magnanimity of a Christian Statesman. The Rannee of Travancore has rejoiced to profit by his counsels; and the result of those counsels has been, that the civil and social condition of her subjects has been rapidly improved; and it will continue to improve, so long as Colonel Munro's advice and plans shall be acted on.[26]

Conditions in the state deteriorated during subsequent decades, leading the Governor-General of India, Lord Dalhousie (1812–1860), to threaten in no uncertain terms annexation unless "averted by timely and judicious reforms".[27] As Jeffrey has argued, the level of intervention in Princely internal affairs increased following the Indian Rebellion or Mutiny of 1857.[28] Ramusack suggests that in the case of Travancore the major reforms during the 1860s and 1870s were due to the conjunction of a "sympathetic young ruler (Ayilyam Tirunal), an able young Dewan (T. Madhava Rao), and a new British resident (F.N. Maltby)".[29] The reforms included collection of land revenue that enabled the state to pay off its debts, namely a hefty annual subsidy to the British; establishment of a public works department, which built roads that encouraged internal trade and provided alternative wage labour for lower castes; bureaucratization of the administration;[30] and the establishment of state-supported schools that linked government service to educational qualifications.[31] Like Napier before him, the Liberal member of parliament in Britain, Sir Henry Fawcett (1833–1884) bestowed praise on the driving force behind the reform measures, Dewan Madava Rao, whom he described in a speech in the House of Commons as "the Turgot of India", who had found Travancore "in the lowest stage of degradation" in 1849 and "left it a Model State" in 1872.[32] The Maharaja's own praise of his first minister was no less exuberant: "What Pericles did for Athens, what Cromwell did for England, that Madava Row did for Travancore."[33] Wider British economic interests and precepts of good modern governance were in harmony, then, with Princely endeavours to please the supreme power in South Asia lest Travancore might be fully integrated into the British Empire.

Late nineteenth-century medical reforms and social stratification

The medical reforms undertaken by "Travancore's Cromwell" during this period received many positive commentaries. Edinburgh-trained Dr Aeneas Mcleod Ross (1837–1886),[34] *darbar* physician and principal medical officer of Travancore, noted that, "As might be expected from the liberal support afforded by His Highness the Maha Raja's Government, the work of the Medical Department for [1870/1] shows a very material increase over all past years."[35] The number of patients treated in hospitals had risen significantly, from 46,019 in 1869 to 66,757 in 1870. This was partly due, Ross explained, to the continued prevalence of a cholera epidemic, but was also accounted for by him by "the increased diligence and faithfulness in their work of the Medical Subordinates and to an extending confidence in them on the part of the Public".[36] Despite these improvements, Ross referred to their current limitations and the scope for further reforms, not just in Travancore, but also in British India:

> It has been affirmed that "the state of the Medical [art] and of the medical health, is no doubt one of the surest tests of a nation's civilization". If this be so, Travancore, like the rest of India, has much room for progress.[37]

There was indeed still much to be done in both British India and in Travancore if modern medical and sanitary provision along European lines was envisaged. While commenting on good environmental conditions, such as the climate, Ross pointed out that the region was "afflicted with a high rate of mortality arising from zymotic or preventable diseases", namely 'fevers' and contagious diseases.[38] He pinpointed some of the causes for this: "The occurrence of these is due to an almost total absence of all sanitary precautions or observances both as regards the state and as regards the individual."[39] He contended that, "The higher Officials of the state are fully alive to the importance of these, but they are totally ignored practically, if not also theoretically, by the minor Officials and by the people at large."[40] Given this apparent lack of awareness amongst subaltern officials and the wider public, he suggested that changes ought to be introduced, but only gradually:

> Little in the way of improvement can be done until their cooperation either voluntary or compulsory is secured. It would I fear be useless to expect any benefit from sweeping measures of sanitary reform. Any measures of the kind to be productive of permanent good must be gradually introduced. The pressure of them will then not be felt, materially at least, and in time the people will be prepared for further progress.[41]

Ross appears to have appreciated that rash developments would engender public resentment against the resulting higher taxes and make them less culturally acceptable. He did however suggest immediate action in regard to the water supply outside temples in order to prevent its contamination by worshippers.[42] These measures, he argued, were possible without interfering "with the liberty of individuals".[43] As Mishra, Johnson and Khalid, and others have shown in regard to vaccination campaigns and sanitary control measures at pilgrimage sites in British India and other areas, the perceived congruence of innovations with cultural sentiments was a vital aspect in their acceptability.[44] Resistance was likely if force was used and the impression of interference in religious customs raised. Unlike some of his colleagues in British Indian provinces, Ross appears to have been particularly perceptive about these issues. He engaged in public awareness initiatives, giving lectures "to arouse the attention of the educated classes to the subject and secure their co-operation" and preparing "a little work on Physiology and Hygiene . . . for the use in the schools".[45] These were aimed at "interesting the people and gradually smoothing the way to the adoption of decided measures in the direction of sanitary reform".[46] Within his wider scheme of consciousness raising Ross promised "shortly to submit propositions for the gradual introduction of sanitary measures commencing as an experimental measure at the capital".[47]

Resistance to medical and sanitary innovations had been observed in, but was not restricted to, the majority Hindu population. As the London Missionary Society member Samuel Mateer (1835–1893) pointed out in 1883, in an overly generalizing way, "The Muhammedans" were not readily inclined to accept Western medical and spiritual intervention. In fact, Mateer considered their conduct during the cholera epidemic of 1875 "deplorable".[48] Apparently, "they stubbornly refused to take medicine, on the plea that their Koran prescribes no remedy for cholera".[49] What is more, they

> sacrificed cocks, goats, and even young bulls, tumultuously calling upon evil spirits whom they considered to be the cause of the plague, to abandon their dwellings and to repair to those of the heathens or Christians. When this proved ineffectual, the males of the village joined together, and bawled out simultaneously a prayer.[50]

If we were to trust Mateer's accounts, then inter-faith relationships were marked by mutual feelings of condescension and distrust.

Statistics provided by Ross for 1870/1 on the social background of in- and out-patients at the Charity and the Civil Hospital in the capital reveal a preponderance of lower and outcastes in the former amongst the in-patients, and of higher castes, in particular Nair, amongst both in- and out-patients in the latter.[51] This is of course only to be expected, given that the civil hospital was then brand new, having been established just six years earlier, while the charity hospital had been founded much less recently, in 1838.[52]

Table 5.1 Charity Hospital. Caste of patients treated, 1870/1.[53]

	In-patients	Out-patients
Numboory Brahmins	–	2
Pandy Brahmins	1	893
Castes between Nairs and Brahmins	16	1,165
Nairs	85	1,025
Artizan Classes	21	84
Lower Castes	31	212
Outcastes	121	8
Mahomedans	9	84
East Indians	–	14
Native Christians	49	48
Outcaste Christians	15	–
	348	3,535

Table 5.1 illustrates that caste precepts of social distance had a considerable impact on the social composition of hospital patients. In the Charity Hospital the majority of in-patients came from lower- and outcaste families, making higher-caste groups disinclined to stay on the same premises. There were 167 in-patients clearly identified as lower or outcastes, in contrast to just 102 higher castes (if artisans, "Native Christians" and Muslims are excluded from the calculation as their position in the caste hierarchy is difficult to gauge). In contrast, the proportion amongst out-patients was drastically reversed, with 3,085 patients being classed as higher and 220 as lower and out caste. Although "all castes and classes shared in the benefits" of the institution, as Ross would have it, they did so in very different ways and to varying extents.[54] However, whether the differing numbers of in- and out-patients signifies socially discriminative admission and access policies, or particular social communities' health-related behaviours and choices is difficult to ascertain.

As Table 5.2 shows the social composition of in- and out-patients in the Civil Hospital was overall in favour of the clearly identified higher castes, with just 289 lower-/outcaste compared to 564 higher-caste in-patients, and 2,498 lower-/outcaste in contrast to 4,051 higher-caste out-patients. Here a detached ward was also made available for Brahmin women.[55]

In contrast to the Charity Hospital, Europeans too frequented this institution, as in- but mostly as out-patients. Menon suggests in the *Kerala District Gazetteer* of 1962 that, "In those days only very poor people afflicted with incurable

Table 5.2 Civil Hospital. Caste of patients treated, 1870/1[56]

	In-patients	Out-patients
Numboory Brahmins	5	192
Malayalum Brahmins	44	275
Pandy Brahmins	66	411
Caste between Brahmins and Nairs	41	265
Nair	408	2908
Artizan Class	38	308
Eloovahs	115	1597
Outcastes	165	609
Mahomedans	44	275
Europeans	5	173
East Indians	6	515
Native Christians	28	655
Outcaste Christians	18	292
	974	8,475

diseases came in as in-patients."[57] Although caste does not necessarily equate with wealth, Menon's contention may not be entirely accurate. Caste-specific services and certain privileges for higher castes were retained even during the 1930s when significant reforms had been introduced by government. For example, during the Murajapam festival in 1935/6, it was decreed that the Fort Hospital ought to "accommodate Namboodiri patients" on a temporary basis and three Brahmin compounders alongside two Brahmin ward attendants were appointed to attend to them.[58] What the effect of these measures would have been for those patients who found themselves temporarily deprived of medical care was not reflected on by the authorities, even at a time when sensitivities towards caste discrimination were pronounced.[59] The authorities' measures on the ground were clearly not always in line with official declarations on caste reform.

As well as caste, gender and cultural sensitivities came to the fore in the lying-in or maternity hospital, which, according to Ross "continues, although very slowly, to grow in favour and usefulness".[60] Only 63 women were admitted in 1870, of whom 25 were high and 38 lower caste; there were also a total of 77 out-patients. Giving birth in an institution instead of at home was clearly not quite as acceptable to both higher and lower caste women as general medical treatment had become in the capital once the Civil Hospital was opened. Even towards the turn of the century, when there were 327 in- and 9,853 out-patients, it was reported that, "Women of respectable families are reluctant to go to hospitals for treatment and would prefer to be treated by one of their sex in their own houses."[61]

There were also the Palace Hospital (468 patients treated in 1870) and the Huzzoor Cutcherry [Secretariat] Hospital (582 patients treated),[62] as well as a dispensary "opened in connection with the Jail Hospital", which was intended to "afford greater convenience to the inhabitants of the Fort" and provided relief for 83 patients.[63] A hospital for the Nayar Brigade had been sanctioned in 1835.[64] People in the capital and the military were therefore comparatively well provided for as far as Western-style medical provision was concerned. Ross did not refer to the Ayurveda Department that existed alongside the Western-style Medical Department. The rulers of Travancore were careful to lend their support to both strands of medicine lest they might upset particular influential communities amongst their subjects and so jeopardize the continued stability of Princely power.

Between 1864 and 1890, medical provision was gradually extended beyond the capital. Sites for the construction of hospitals at Kottayam, Changanacherry (Changanassery), Alleppey, Mavelikkara, and Quilon (Kollam) were identified.[65] In 1866, the "extension of means of medical aid in the country" was discussed alongside other measures such as "poverty schools", a higher branch of education, and the establishment of a lunatic asylum at Trivandrum.[66] Developments in subsequent years included a hospital at Padmanabhapuram (later transferred to Thakalay/Thakkalai) and at Peermade hillstation.[67] However, by the 1870s only a few "out station hospitals" and medical facilities attached to public works corps were available in areas outside the capital. These included Mavalikaray (324 in-patients; 7,735 out-patients treated during 1870); Cottayam (605; 5,835); Allepey (78; 2,787); Parachallay (237; 4,206); and Pulpanabhapooram (313; 4,089).[68] Shencottay (Sengottai) had a "native building" and did not admit in-patients, while new facilities were opened at Quilon in 1870 (306; 4,069), and new ones were in progress at Shertallay and Nagercoil, though only old 'native', traditional-style buildings were available here.[69] Hospitals attached to public works projects included Peermade (359 treated), Workallay Barrier (1,380), Meenmooty (261), and Ariyencavoo Pass (722).[70] Cardamom Hill, which consisted of thick rain forest and was dedicated to cardamom cultivation, had a medical facility that treated 84 people during 1870. There were also jail hospitals at Quilon, Alleppey, and Nagercoil.

With the boom in tea and coffee cultivation from the 1870s onwards, regular grants were provided by government for the medical care of planters at the Planter's Hospital at Ashambi.[71] Sanatoria were established at hill stations such as Ponmudi.[72]

A similar range of initiatives continued to be undertaken throughout the 1880s and 1890s, when postal and telegraph services were provided and road construction was in full swing, enabling better communication between the main towns and affording access to the rich natural resources of the remote areas. Medical duties and who was entitled to treatment became increasingly more clearly circumscribed. For example, it was decreed in 1884 that officers' servants were not entitled to free medical attendance by *sirkar* or government medical officers.[73] However, there was emphasis during the 1880s and 1890s on the establishment of dispensaries that allowed a greater number of out-patients to be treated.[74] Even medical scholarships for women were considered and rules laid down regarding women's eligibility to apply for them.[75] Finally, in 1896, the constitution of a Medical Board was discussed and the Medical Department re-organized, drawing together the varied medical developments initiated throughout the nineteenth century.[76]

Still, higher castes seem to have profited disproportionately from the reform initiatives, as is suggested by the strong criticism from some, especially missionaries. Reverend Samuel Mateer, for example, bemoaned this phenomenon in 1883 in regard to the educational reforms undertaken during the previous two decades. He noted

> Certainly the Annual Reports of the Administration of Travancore for the last twenty years show a highly admirable increase of attention to higher education, and of expenditure upon it which reflects great credit on the Government, yet we cannot forget that nearly all the effort and most of the expenditure have been on behalf of the higher castes, who really have it in their power to help themselves did they desire to do so, while the lower castes are left almost untouched by the present system of education.[77]

Mateer agreed with the assessment of the reforms published in *The Western Star* (established in Cochin in 1860), that considered the expenditure on Brahmans in Travancore "altogether disproportionate to their numbers, and unfair to other elements of the population".[78] Not unsurprisingly, he noted that, "The Christians strongly object to this expenditure of the public funds". However, discontent was also rife amongst other groups that felt disadvantaged:

> The low castes have been sorely oppressed by the temple services; and the Nayars, who have had some little pleasure and benefit from this expenditure, are more and more indulging in complaints of sacerdotal pretensions, and beginning to rebel against their inequitable exclusion on various occasions. Intelligent Sudras are far from being content with the present state of things.[79]

As this evidence shows, educational and medical reforms during this period tended to be focused on the capital and major provincial towns, on the alleviation of sickness amongst labourers connected with infrastructural and plantation projects, and displayed a distinct higher-caste bias.

Medical reforms and funding priorities

The costs of the health reforms were considerable, as Ross pointed out in 1870/1:

> as might be expected from the liberal support afforded by His Highness the Maharaja's Government, the work of the Medical Department for the year [1870] shows a very material increase over all past years. In the preceding year the total number of patients treated in the Travancore Hospitals . . . amounted to 46,019, while during [1870] it reached the much higher figure of 66,757.[80]

The question then arises of how much H.R.H. the Maharaja of Travancore was willing to spend on the medical department in his state (see Table 5.3). How did support for medicine figure in contrast to other state expenditure in 1870/1?

Table 5.3 Charges for medical department, 1870/1[81]

Salaries of the medical establishment	33,401
Medical supplies	46,840
Dieting and contingencies	26,769
Vaccination Department	10,144
	Rs 1,17,154

If the figures for medical provision during the 1870s displayed in the above Table are compared to other departmental expenses, such as the construction of the Quilon and Shencotta roads, which were so important for the spice trade during this period, it can be seen that they are roughly equal. They amounted to a total of Rs 1,13,000.[82] How we evaluate this fact is more complex. After all, whether the medical department compares well with the expenditure on transport infrastructure is a matter for socio-political and economic debate, particularly if we are inclined to take into account which social groups gained from the different measures. The analysis is no less complex if medical and other social welfare institutions – the chief minister's "surest tests of a nation's civilization" – are looked at in relation to the state's overall expenses.

Table 5.4 Expenditure for 1870/71. Dewan's Report on the Finances, 10.11.1871[83]

The Davasom or religious institutions	5,52,827
Ootooperah or charitable institutions	3,05,950
The palace	4,99,549
Huzzoor Cutcherry and other civil establishments	5,65,867
Judicial establishment	1,32,956
Police establishment	1,57,415
Nair troops	1,77,597
Elephant and horse establishment	65,696
Education, science, and art	1,23,244
Pensions	1,21,517
Public works	11,68,728
Cost and charges of goods sold, &c.	4,13,969
Contingent charges	1,96,593[*]
Subsidy to British Indian government	8,10,652
Total	52,92,560

Year's Income: 52,44,472

According to Table 5.4 it appears that the Medical Department was funded on a similar level to the police, judicial, and education departments and that it certainly received more financial support than the "Elephant and Horse Establishment". On the other hand, within the wider scheme of things, spending for medical provision was not especially prioritized during this period. The palace and government services as well as religious institutions – all of them vital to the maintenance of the ruler's prestige, power, and influence – received more attention. Meanwhile the lion's share of state income was used to support public works and a substantial sum was given to the British colonial government.[84] (A decade later, in 1879, the total cost of the Medical Department was reported to have been Rs 50,000 plus contingent charges of Rs 20,000. Medical stores were valued at Rs 30,000 and vaccinations at Rs 10,000, which brought the total expenditure of the Department to Rs 1,10,000.[85])

The role of missionaries and caste reform

As Kooiman and Cox have shown, missionaries had an important role to play in regard to changing social conditions in Travancore.[86] They campaigned for social reform, were frequently ardent critics of social injustices, and even used their influence (as in the case of Charles Grant and John Munro) to press for intervention by the British. Missionaries were tolerated and to a certain extent supported by the indigenous rulers in the early nineteenth century. During Munro's time in the second decade of the nineteenth century, the Prussian Lutheran William Ringeltaube received grants to spread the gospel amongst lower- and outcaste Hindus, although conversions were rare.[87] According to Hacker, early missionaries were well aware of the slow progress in terms of real conversions to Christian beliefs, as the poor availed themselves of the services provided by the missions without changing their creed.[88]

During the second half of the nineteenth century, Reverend Mateer, the outspoken critic of government's measures of reform, put the situation as he then perceived it in a nutshell: "The system of Government in Travancore practically consists of two benevolent despotisms, the Native and the British, the one acting as a counteraction to the other."[89] The Princely government lent support to some missionary initiatives, such as by providing grants-in-aid for Neyyoor mission hospital in 1853, 1868, 1869, 1871, 1874, and 1875.[90] This kind of provision was in line with charitable donations by the Princely state for medical relief of Indians in British provinces. Examples include the lying-in hospital in the 'Black Town', or Indian part, of Madras; educational projects such as the 'female school' in Calcutta (Kolkata); and famine relief in Bengal.[91] However, Mateer still had an axe to grind with both the British and the Princely governments as neither consistently and wholeheartedly approved of what they considered to be missionaries' interference in social affairs and customs. Mateer complained:

> We hear of petty officious interference with missionary preachers, driving off people quietly assembled to listen or to obtain medical treatment, threatening with dismissal those who wish to receive tracts, driving Pulayars [outcastes, previously enslaved] off the road, and so forth. One head constable arrested and locked up a Mission catechist of the highest character and standing.[92]

Missionaries such as Mateer expressed strong views on the whole range of reforms that were undertaken during the 1860s and 1870s; including those pertaining to land ownership and revenue collection. In regard to revenue reform, Mateer suggested that it should include "a separation of the duties connected with the management of the extensive religious and charitable establishments from purely revenue and magisterial duties", as this would be "a most essential and urgent item of needed reform".[93] The land reforms of 1865, which conferred land ownership on state tenants, had made land saleable and allowed Travancore's untouchables (Ezhavas) to become smallholders.[94] Nevertheless, while private land ownership came to be spread amongst many more castes than had hitherto been the case, the state remained in charge of the majority of land, with comparatively low taxes demanded from tenants.[95] The commodification of land was vital to the establishment of a new agricultural order that attracted future outside investment and replaced the exploitation of agricultural labour on the basis of caste with the order created by the invisible hand of the market.[96]

Ezhava communities, largely made up of agricultural workers considered untouchable, were particularly successful in lobbying government and benefited most from land reforms. They did not convert to Christianity (unlike the lower caste Shanars), but used conversion as a threat to accelerate social reform. Gaining education also raised expectations amongst high-status Nayars and Syrian Christians.[97] Caste inequalities included lower caste women being forbidden from covering their breasts and untouchables being prevented from using temples and roads. Caste reform movements towards the late nineteenth century, while still anchored in the Hindu belief system, nevertheless emphasized the idea that caste itself was irrational and unscientific, and hence rejected religion-based exploitation and social hierarchy.[98] Such explicit reference to Western notions of social equality and science did however not imply reformers' subservience to British supremacy in South Asia. From the early twentieth century in particular, social reformers expressed anti-colonial sentiments, no longer being bamboozled by the ideology of the mythical 'British sense for fairness and just government' that apparently excused colonial hegemony.[99]

At the same time, Christianity constituted an escape from the social constraints of the caste system for disempowered and exploited communities. Consequently, the influence of missionaries increased steadily as conversion rates rose over the course of the nineteenth century. Welfare and education provision for the lowest strata of the population were a challenge for a monarchy, whose perceived legitimacy depended partly on its reputation for *dharmabhumi*: preservation of the welfare of its people in the realms of law and religious duty, as well as concern with the socio-moral order of the cosmos.[100] As Kooiman argues, during the nineteenth century the missions and government settled into a kind of division of charitable impulse, with the former being given public grants to provide for the lowest castes and untouchables, and the government establishing separate facilities for the higher orders of society.[101] However, in relation to education, Kawashima notes not only the emergent dynamics in the relationship between missions and the state but also the peculiar coalition of interests between high and low castes, both of which came to demand the establishment of government-run 'schools for all' that did not require them to leave Hinduism or claim spiritual conversion.[102]

As such, the greatest success of the missions could be considered the impetus that they provided towards universal education delivered by government at a time when Hindu sentiments were heightened yet traditional religious schools were considered outmoded.[103]

Desai emphasizes that the roles of Christian missions and of the state need to be set against the wider regional context, noting that "the reforms were a preemptive response to British proximity and the threat of annexation as well as the [perceived] threat of mass conversions to Christianity."[104] Arguably, this led to Travancore having one of the highest literacy rates amongst both Princely states and British provinces by the 1930s. British Burma (37 percent of ages five and over) and Princely Cochin (34 percent) led, but Travancore (29 percent) was well ahead of Princely Baroda (21 percent); British Bengal, British Madras and Princely Mysore (all eleven percent); British Bihar and Orissa (five percent); and the Princely Bihar and Orissa states (four percent).[105] However, despite modernization and the emergence of new notions of citizenship and the duty of the state, considerable caste-based inequalities remained. Furthermore, the fluctuations of a market-based economy and, according to Desai, Travancore's dependence on the export market, created unprecedented unemployment and risk of famines.[106] This gave ample scope for, and indeed necessitated, prestige-enhancing measures of welfare relief that could counteract what Juergen Habermas referred to as a "legitimation crisis".

Religious welfare institutions and Brahmin privileges

As in all south Indian states, religious patronage and leadership were vital aspects of Indian governance.[107] According to ancient Sanskrit texts, such as the *Arthashastra*, rulers were meant to mediate in cases of caste, social, and religious disputes. Dirks has shown that this role implied that political power was vital to the ways caste boundaries were drawn.[108] Good kings were supposed to provide support for religious institutions and patronize scholars; this was part of the process by which Princely rule was legitimized and ennobled. King Marthanda Varma (1706–1758) had dedicated Travancore to an incarnation of Vishnu (Lord Padmanabha), enabling his successors to conceive themselves both symbolically and constitutionally as servants of the deity, stabilizing their rule by adding further clout to their position.[109] Although Travancore introduced a legislative council with appointed members as early as 1888 and an elected consultative assembly in 1904, as in other Princely states, these assemblies initially had an advisory function only.[110]

State expenditure on "*devasoms*" (Devaswom, religious institutions) and on "*oottooperahs*" (Ootupara, charitable inns for pilgrims) attest to the strong link between Hindu religion and kingship in Travancore. As Table 5.4 (see page 93), reveals, Devaswom and Ootupara received the sums of Rs 552,827 and Rs 305,950 in 1870/1, respectively. These were the highest items of expenditure after the palace and public administration (Rs 499,549 and Rs 565,867, respectively), public works (Rs 1,168,728), and the state's subsidy to the British Indian government (Rs 810,652). Together they amounted to nearly six times as much as the medical department had to rely on.

Yet intriguingly the upkeep of Devaswoms was not, according to Dewan Nagam Aiya (1850–1917), considered part of the Maharaja's duties until 1811/12. Aiya suggested that, "The State had no concern with the management of any temples before the year [1811–1812], when the landed property of 378 temples was assumed by the State and the management taken over."[111] This takeover apparently happened during the time of Colonel Munro, "the Resident-Dewan".[112] The lands formerly owned by the temples "were leased out to the ryots [cultivators] on the tenure known as *Sirkar Pattom* [government lease]".[113] Some 1,171 temples without land were "also assumed either before or at that date".[114] At least in regard to temples, the state's role was not simply and exclusively part of a supposedly age-old tradition, but a result of British interests and influence. This new "permanent settlement" affected the "expenditure, establishments, the routine of ceremonies, rules for the management, &c.".[115] Hinting at the British and subsequent Princely twin rationales of social enlightenment and fiscal profits, Nagam Aiya argued:

> This important measure carried out after the military occupation of these territories by the British Government has undoubtedly done much good by rescuing from capricious and corrupt management a vast extent of valuable real property estimated to yield a revenue of nearly 4½ lakhs of rupees and placing it under the systematic control of the Government of the country.[116]

The expenditure was calculated to be offset by the income, but it seems that the figures did not add up consistently.[117] In his report of 1873/4, Dewan Sashia Sastri (A. Seshayya Sastri, 1828–1903, Dewan: 1872–1880) claimed that:

> The interest of Government in respect of these institutions is for the most part only that of a Trustee, and even were it otherwise, this State will be bound as every other country in the world does to maintain a Church establishment out of public revenue.[118]

A modern rationale was used to offset any potential objections to the Princely government deriving financial gains from religious establishments. In addition to any gains or losses, the state achieved control over, and political allegiance from, the groups affiliated to the temples. The total number of people affiliated with the religious establishments in this way was considerable: 4,455 in the 1870s.[119] Each temple had: officiating priests (*shanties*), a manager, *pillay* (accountant), shroff or cash-keeper, storekeeper, light keeper, sweepers, four to eight Nair women to sweep the premises, musicians and, in southern districts, also dancing girls. In a gesture designed to pre-empt any criticisms of the extraordinary expenses that the maintenance of these institutions incurred, Sashia Sastri contended:

> So far as the people are concerned it is to them a source of the deepest gratification in a religious point, and to thousands of the poor of all classes and creeds, they are the means of furnishing a subsistence.[120]

Nevertheless, the system connected with Devaswoms, including the custom of selling on at cut-market prices temple offerings of rice was clearly controversial, as the Dewan admitted: "universal concurrence is not to be expected of course".[121]

The maintaining of Ootuparas from public funds was even more contentious, but similarly ennobling for the Maharaja in ideological terms. It ensured support from the group that most benefitted from them: Brahmans and in the capital Nairs and, to a certain extent, Sudras. Ootuparas were feeding stations or pilgrims' inns "intended chiefly for Brahmins" and located in the capital and along the main road from Aramboly in the south to Parur in the north.[122] They were strategically placed so that a travelling Brahmin would never go without food the whole way.[123] The largest of these inns was in the capital, known as the Agrasala and "intended to feed all comers both day and night".[124] The Agrasala benefited from the extensive corridors and galleries of Padmanabhaswamy Pagoda for use as dining halls. The number fed daily at breakfast and supper amounted to about 1,500 people of the Brahman caste on each occasion. The 103 staff members affiliated with this establishment were also entitled to receive free meals, as were "Several thousands of Nayars and other Sudras for services connected with the Pagoda and the Agrasala".[125] In addition, uncooked rice was "distributed to Brahmins who [did] not eat in the Agrasala, and to non Brahmins attached to Palace, by Royal favour".[126] Overall the amount allocated to the 40 or so Ootuparas of all kinds (including the feeding of cows with fresh grass) was Rs 406,641 by 1903/4. This community-specific charity compares starkly with the expenditure for the Medical Department that was by then meant to provide for people of all walks of life in the state.

However, while Western medicine was part of modernity and relatively new, the *raison d'être* of Ootuparas linked in with the trope of the Maharaja's benevolent rule or *dharma raj*, as evoked by the Maharaja's speech during the opening of the Civil Hospital in Trivandrum in 1865: "For time out of mind, charity has been regarded by Travancore as one of the cardinal duties of the state. Its reputation as Dhurma Raj is familiar to all India."[127] As we have seen, even the Revd. Samuel Mateer referred to Travancore as "the land of charity", using the term as the title of one of his books.[128] Ootuparas were justified on the basis of supposedly 'ancient tradition'. They were said to have existed well before the middle of the eighteenth century, when Maharaja Marthanda Varma (1706–1758) and his Dewan, Ramayyan Dalwa (Rama Iyen; ?-1756), established "modern Travancore" by annexing smaller principalities.[129] On ceding their sovereignty, the former rulers expressly stipulated that "you shall protect the people, the Gods and the Brahmins according to previous custom."[130] Travancore duly followed this injunction, dedicating large sums to the support of Brahmins in particular. Sir Madava Rao (?1828–1891) argued in 1871 that "apart from such obligations the Maharajahs as Sovereigns of a purely Hindu State have always regarded it as a religious duty to keep up such institutions."[131] Perhaps more to the point of the balance of power, such observation of religious duty and preservation of established customs and privileges helped avert potential unrest in the freshly annexed regions and secure the loyalty of influential communities.

Successful maharajas and Dewans catered for and invoked both the traditional and the modern, following what the one-time Governor of Madras, Lord (Francis) Napier (1819–1898), had referred to as a "judicious and prudent middle way".[132] This was seen by him to ensure the "confidence" of their people while meeting the "discriminating expectation of a progressive age" and hence of the British supreme power in South Asia.[133]

Indigenous medicine and Vaidyasalas

The support of Ootuparas and Devaswoms bowed to religious tradition – however ancient or recently invented – pleasing and appeasing Brahmins, in particular. In the field of medicine, too, successive rulers and their Dewans sponsored the indigenous alongside the Western sector. Increased provision for Western-style medicine was therefore consistently complemented by financial resources for traditional medical approaches. Ayurvedic medicine was the main traditional system that received support by the state. Aiya reported that grants were provided on a regular basis from the late 1880s:

> With a view to give a stimulus to the study of Native medicine in which the bulk of the population, especially in the rural parts, have great faith, and as an encouragement to Native practitioners, His Highness the Maharajah was pleased to sanction grants-in-aid to a few select Native Vydians to enable them to dispense medicines to the poor free of charge.[134]

Who the "select" practitioners were is not discussed by Aiya. In Travancore practitioners from different caste communities practised Ayurvedic medicine. Panikkar notes that Ayurveda was not a monopoly of the upper castes and hence not limited to practitioners belonging to *ashtavaidyan* upper-caste families and their disciples.[135] In fact, it is reasonable to assume that the majority of doctors with an Ayurvedic frame of reference would have belonged to the lower and even untouchable castes, reflecting the background of their patient base. The popularity of Narayana Guru (*c.* 1856–1928), the important social reformer of the Ezhavas (a low-caste community considered as untouchable by the Nambudiri Brahmins), was, as Pannikar argues, "built around his knowledge of medicine and ability to cure diseases".[136]

When, during another set of reforms in 1895/6, medical grants were sanctioned in support of hospitals and dispensaries, in order to "encourage medicine by private agency under organised control", Vaidyasalas (Ayurvedic in- or out-patient dispensaries), too, received funding on a regular basis.[137] At this point, it is likely that the "committee" of "two leading native physicians appointed by Government, to whom all applications for grants were to be referred and whose duty was to advise government on all professional and other matters connected with the *Vaidyasalas*" were recruited from high-caste *ashtavaidyan* lineages.[138] The following year, the grants-in-aid to Vaidyasalas were "improved and extended and rules passed prescribing the conditions of the grants and the duties and responsibilities

of the applicants for the same".[139] Arguably, this was the time when the param-
eters of what was to be considered legitimate Ayurvedic practice became formally
circumscribed by means of central state authority and those who did not fulfil the
stipulated criteria were marginalized and considered as backward and unqualified
'quacks' or heterodox doctors.

By 1903/4, the number of Vaidyasalas supported by government grants had
risen from 28 in 1896/7 to 68.[140] At this stage, 120,626 patients were treated in
these Ayurvedic dispensaries, amounting to nearly 20 percent of the total treated
by state-sponsored medical institutions.[141] Dewan Aiya noted: "The native system
of treatment known as *Ashtangahridayam* is slowly reviving under the encouragement now extended by His Highness' Government."[142] He was well aware of
the fact that state-funded institutions and the elite Ayurveda practised in them
provided medical services for but a small percentage of the population: "But as
a matter of fact the proportion of the sick that resort to the Sirkar [government]
medical institutions is only very small."[143] The majority of the people, he pointed
out, were "still resorting only to the native *Vaidyans* of the rural villages".[144]
There was a considerable divide between "the recognised *Vaidyans*", who maintained Vaidyasalas, and the "hundreds of native *Vaidyans* practising throughout
the country".[145] The latter, he contended "do not care to preserve a record of their
practice" and hence "the actual statistics of the sick treated under the native system are not available".[146]

The number of patients treated in the few officially registered, funded and cen-
trally controlled Vaidyasalas and European-style institutions had increased significantly, and, as Aiya suggested, the Travancorean was "more considerately treated
in this respect by the Native government than at any period".[147] However, it still
was the case that

> to the large numbers of the working classes [state-funded institutions] are
> beyond reach, not on account of the indifference or unwillingness of the
> medical authorities to treat them, but owing more to their ignorance and
> their general apathy. In the case of the well-to-do classes, by far the largest
> proportion of them believe in the efficacy of their 'native' medicines and
> the native system of doctoring known as Ashtangahridayam. The bulk of
> the Namburi [Nambudiri] Brahmins as well as the Sudras, and a good many
> of the middle classes follow the prescriptions of these Ashtangahridayam
> Vydians.[148]

What was more, according to Aiya, "Many of these are mere quacks, but the
popular faith in them remains yet unshaken."[149] The kind of services provided at
Vaidyasalas were clearly not representative of the common practices available to
and considered acceptable and efficacious by the wider population, in particular
in areas outside the urban centres. There was of course, as the Dewan noted, the
select group of Nambudiri doctors who "trace their medical profession to the time
of Parasurama", an avatar of Vishnu, from whom, as the foundation myth suggested, their ancestors received their "secrets of the science" directly.[150] However,

as Aiya was well aware, the field of medicine was overwhelmingly characterized by plurality:

> numerous Sudra [lower caste] doctors too well versed in Ashtangahridayam all over the country, and some Iluva [low caste], Syrian Christian and also Mahomedan vydians are known to claim proficiency in the native methods of treatment. There is no Kara [village] without its vydian, and in thickly-peopled villages, old women act the part of vydians in every-day ailments and the part of midwives in obstetric cases.[151]

Two important issues arise from this situation in regard to the financial support received by specific branches of medical practice and the extent to which these catered for but a fraction of the population. First, government spent by 1903/4 Rs 410,000 on the medical and sanitary departments, which amounted to about four percent of the total income of the year.[152] This, Aiya held, attested to a "liberal and enlightened policy" and compared "favourably with any other State or Province in India".[153] However, as in other regions, and as highlighted by Aiya himself, the majority of the population did not profit from these outlays, as it did not have access to or was disinclined to make use of the kind of medical services – Western and indigenous – provided by the state.

Second, as was the case also in other regions in South Asia, a great variety of practitioners from different social and educational backgrounds and with varied knowledge bases populated the field of medicine in Travancore. As before the advent of European influence in the region, a medical hierarchy, mirroring prevalent caste divisions, prevailed. However, from the late nineteenth century the medical pecking order became increasingly formalized and circumscribed by means of central state regulation. This enshrined the privileged position of particular practitioners groups in terms of Western criteria of professionalized practice, training, and efficacy. An example of this is the founding of an Ayurveda Pathasala or training school in 1889 at East Fort at Trivandrum, offering a four-year training course,[154] which was extended to five years in 1917,[155] eventually leading, in 1918, to a further revision "on up-to-date and scientific lines in order to suit modern requirement", with the integration of physiology and anatomy into the curriculum. This led to the status of the Pathasala being raised to that of Government Ayurveda College in 1921.[156] In 1928, the proposition to give state recognition to qualified and expert Vaidyas was sanctioned, sealing the process by which a particular approach of Ayurveda became professionalized along Western lines.[157] Minority practices such as homoeopathy and Unani, too, became officially accredited and regulated. The former approach was introduced in 1906 by Dr M.N. Pillai.[158] A "Unani Vaidyasala" was established, situated at the cantonment in Trivandrum and, according to Menon, it treated 300 patients per month.[159]

The need to regulate the training and practice of Ayurveda was also considered pressing in neighbouring British-ruled Calicut, where the eminent high-caste Ayurvedic practitioner P.S. Variar (1869–1944) established a Vaidyasala and workshop for the production of Ayurvedic drugs in 1902, and a Pathasala in 1917.[160]

Variar initiated in 1902 an association of physicians, the Arya Vaidya Samajam, of which the Maharaja of Travancore was a patron (alongside the ruler of Cochin and the Samuthiri or Zamorin of Calicut). The Samajam's annual conferences became, as Panikkar notes, "big cultural events" that were an "ideational ground of the revitalization movement" in the south west, which aimed at reviving the "once prosperous and increasingly declining Ayurveda", providing training based on the mastery of ancient Sanskrit texts for practitioners and, last but not least "acquaint[ing] the British government about the merits of the indigenous system".[161] Like elite practitioners in Travancore, Variar reconciled the revitalizing agenda with a plea for "a dialogue between eastern and western medicine".[162] Treading a "middle path" was a diplomatic and pragmatic approach in a situation where the British kept a keen and critical eye on developments in their own provinces and in the Princely states.

It was not until 1942/3 when another set of reforms was implemented in the Medical Department and measures were "adopted for preventing the evils that befall the public from treatment by unskilled medical men".[163] The reported "evils" were not restricted to indigenous practitioners; the Medical Practitioners' Bill made it compulsory for doctors of all traditions to register. By 1946/7, 124 applications for registration had been received, with a further 1,767 pending, making a total of 1,891 of which 926 were granted registration.[164] The nature or class of the license was dependent on the practitioner's qualifications and the healthcare facilities made available to patients (see Table 5.5).

Table 5.5 Applications for medical registrations, 1946/7[165]

System	Class A	Class B	Total
Allopathy	78	48	126
Ayurveda	46	466	512
Sidha [Siddha]		221	221
Homoeopathy		57	57
Dentistry		6	6
Unani		4	4
Total			*926*

Regulations were put in place also in regard to the marketing of particular practices. In 1946/6, for example, "a few practitioners" received a warning for having been "found guilty of professional advertisements".[166]

Medical education, too, was focused on during this period, with increased inspection and quality assurance requirements being enforced. While Ayurveda had by this time well-established training schools, the situation was less formalized in regard to Siddha. In fact the Medical Council appointed a new committee in 1946/7 to inspect and report on the working of the "Sidha Vaydia School" conducted by the All Travancore Sidha Vaydia Sanghom at Munchirai. Arrangements there had been subject to complaints about their "inadequacy . . . to impart instruction in medicine".[167] The "absence of qualified teachers" was noted, leading to recommendations that "the diplomas issued by the Sanghom should be removed from the schedule of recognised qualifications for registration" in Siddha.[168] The recognition of Siddha by the central authorities lagged well behind Ayurveda, which had by then enjoyed official government support for several decades, not least in terms of financial subsidies. When rules for professional accreditation were tightened, Ayurveda, as the most prominent indigenous medical practice sponsored by government and the Hindu majority population, had the advantage of its early institutionalization as the main traditional paradigm of healing in Travancore.

Professional state accreditation was important for practitioners intent on setting themselves up in private practice. For example, only "deserving private medical practitioners" received a subvention from government to set up "nursing homes" to relieve congestion in government hospitals, like the one attached to the Sri Ramakrishna Ashram and private dispensary at Vakkom.[169] In order to qualify for support, these places needed to be open for inspection to the Surgeon General; continue practice for five years; be run by a registered medical practitioner; and be located in a rural area, at least six miles away from a government or other allopathic medical institution. Grant-in-aid and private hospitals and dispensaries that provided in-patient accommodation and treated poor patients for free received a subvention of Rs 100 per bed (up to a maximum of Rs 1,500).[170] Professionalization, state accreditation, and inspection applied to all branches of official medical practice from the mid-twentieth century onwards.

Medical provision, government spending, and caste in the twentieth century

What was the state of medical provision in Travancore at the beginning of the twentieth century? By 1904, the Western medical department ran 22 hospitals, 21 dispensaries, five bi-weekly and six weekly dispensaries.[171] The number of out-patients remained, as before, much higher than those of in-patients, namely 615,861 and 15,574, respectively. In addition, 23,319 people were treated by fifteen medical officers on special duty, mostly those engaged in sanitation.[172] There were also eight aided institutions (86,497 patients treated) and 64 Vaidyasalas treating 132,395 patients.[173]

A couple of years later, in 1906/7, expenses for Western and for what was referred to as 'native' medicine amounted to the following:[174]

Hospitals and dispensaries	277,625 Rs
Grants to medical institutions	11,516
Grants to native medical institutions	10,688
Native physicians	4,135
Native medical schools	987
Durbar physicians	25,201

Sanitation, vaccination, town improvement, and rural conservancy received separate funding, namely:[175]

Sanitation	28,354 Rs
Vaccination	18,008
Town improvement	64,026
Rural conservancy	22,985

On the basis of the above figures, it appears that spending on Western medicine and affiliated institutions (i.e. hospitals, dispensaries, aided hospitals and dispensaries) was higher by a factor of 290 than what was given to indigenous medicine. Even the maintenance of the *darbar* physician's establishment amounted to considerably more than was allocated in total for indigenous practitioners. While sanitation arrangements fared better, receiving nearly double the support of indigenous medical establishments, it was similar in order to the *darbar* physician's. The continued elite medicine and urban bias is reflected also in the amounts allocated to town in contrast to rural improvements, namely nearly three times as much for just five urban centres. What is more the Maharaja's tour in 1906 to Madras to meet the Prince and Princess of Wales cost more than the annual expenditure of the sanitation and vaccination establishments combined, namely Rs 55,618![176] In Travancore priorities were clearly set, and they were not altogether in favour of medical and public health improvement when compared to what the royal household considered its due and necessary for the maintenance of its standing in the eyes of the British. As Trollope had noted in relation to the higher orders of society in *Barchester Towers*, due observance of rank and prestige could not be maintained unless the (costly) exterior trappings belonging to it were held in proper esteem.

Extensive sums kept being earmarked also for religious and charitable institutions. As throughout the nineteenth century, this continued to earn Travancore's royalty its reputation as charitable and religiously devout rulers, facilitating the legitimation and continuation of royal power. The support of religious institutions alone cost the state nearly twice as much as all medical establishments – Western and indigenous – and sanitation, vaccination, town improvement, and rural conservancy combined, namely an astounding Rs 901,779 in the case of the former and Rs 463,525 for the latter. Charitable institutions, largely aimed at Brahmins, too, fared better, with an allocation of Rs 510,000, although they were not being catered for quite as generously as the British Government, which received a handsome subsidy of Rs 810,878, nearly double as much as medical and public healthcare! It does not take a political radical to wonder whether state income was fairly and sensibly distributed in the "land of charity". Even charity itself, as we have seen, continued to privilege elite caste groups.

By the mid-1930s, the number of out-patients treated in Western government-sponsored institutions had increased threefold in contrast to the early twentieth century (namely to 1,970,758; 2,223,779 by 1945).[177] In-patient numbers remained roughly the same (56,957; albeit there were considerably more, namely 91,457, in 1945). In addition, there were 13,114 in-patients and 212,664 out-patients who received medical treatment at grant-in-aid institutions.[178] The social composition of the population receiving Western healthcare, in the 1930s and 1940s respectively, is intriguing (see Figure 5.1).

Figure 5.1 Assigned religious affiliation of in- and out-patients treated in Western government-sponsored institutions, in percentage, 1935/6 and 1945/6[179]

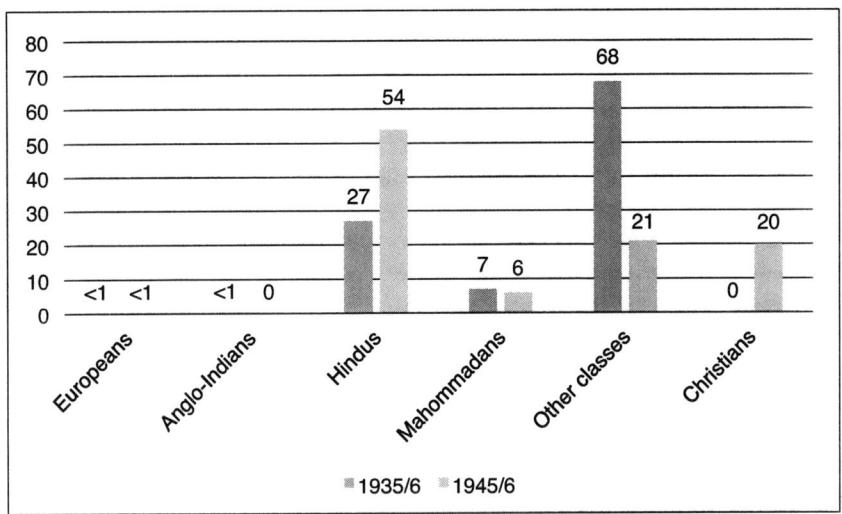

The above Figure highlights a number of issues. Some of these relate to modifications in classification practice concerning particular social groups over the period. Others may be indicative of changes in the accessibility or acceptability of Western-style in- and out-patient institution-based treatment. One of the most conspicuous features is that patients of Christian background were not listed separately until 1945. Judging from the re-arrangement of categories and figures that occurred in 1945, it is likely that earlier on Christians had been subsumed under "other classes".[180] Why was this so? The data are most likely to reflect wider socio-political trends, as lower- and outcaste (Dalit) Hindus converted to Christianity as a potential way out of the injustices of caste discrimination. However, conversion is not necessarily a sudden change due to an individual's spiritual epiphany but may engender personal ambiguities about one's religious identity that might involve a preference to be categorized as "other" in certain circumstances. Hospital admission staff might also be inclined to categorize as "other class" a patient formerly known to them as, or giving the appearance of, an Indian outcaste turned Christian. Institutional statistics in other provinces contrasted "caste Hindus" with "Hindus" to signify people's place in the caste hierarchy.

There were other socio-political issues at stake, too, such as a fear of rising numbers of Christians in a majority Hindu kingdom and the ambition on the part of administrators to exert political correctness at a time when official census nomenclature in relation to oppressed Hindu communities shifted between 'outcastes', 'untouchables', 'Harijans', 'depressed classes', 'external classes', and 'scheduled castes'. For example, in the appendix to the Indian census report of 1931 it was noted that the term 'exterior castes' was adopted "as the most satisfactory alternative to the unfortunate and depressing label 'depressed class' ", which hitherto had been used instead of 'outcastes'.[181] The choice of term was as controversial as the social realities it was to circumscribe, resulting in the decision that depressed or exterior castes were those "contact with whom entails purification on the part of high caste Hindus"; it was not to be employed in the case of Muslims, Christians, and tribes (Adivasis).[182] Such distinctions were bound to lead to confusion, in particular in relation to Dalits-turned-Christians.

Most importantly, the 1920s and 1930s were a period of political upheaval on account of caste movements that had the potential to threaten the stability in the state. Maharaja Sri Chithira Thirunal (1912–1991; reigned: 1924–1949), being counselled by the British and urged by Indian reformers such as Mahatma Gandhi, responded with the passing of the Temple Entry Proclamation in 1931, which signalled a somewhat more progressive attitude towards caste than had hitherto been the case under his predecessors.[183] The Indian Census published in 1931 had revealed that Travancore had the highest proportion of "depressed" or "exterior" castes of all Indian states and British provinces, namely 56 percent of the state's Hindu and 35 percent of the total population.[184] Officially, discrimination on account of caste was not to exist; hospital records reflected this, problems of categorization notwithstanding.

The only group identified in Figure 5.1 that appears to have been unproblematic in terms of its numerical listing were Muslims; their presence amongst in- and out-patients remained of the same order between 1935 and 1945, namely seven and six percent, respectively, roughly identical to their share in overall population numbers as recorded in the census.[185] This is in stark contrast to the Hindu category on the one hand and the "other classes" rubric on the other, which increased, for the former, from 27 percent in 1935 to 54 percent in 1945, and, for the latter, decreased from 68 percent to 21 percent, with the new "Christian" heading identifying 20 percent. Intriguingly, the census data stipulated, for 1935, 27 percent caste and 35 percent outcaste Hindus and, for 1945, 52 percent Hindus and seven percent "external" castes. The census data for Christians were the same in 1935 and 1945, namely 32 percent (in contrast to the 20 percent listed in the hospital statistics in 1945).

Preconceptions of race had previously led to the separate listing of Europeans and those of mixed Euro-Indian background, irrespective of religion. This was common practice in the all-India census, too. Notwithstanding European racial prejudice, social segregation was not in principle anathema to high-caste Indians who considered Europeans ritually polluting. As the end of the British *Raj* came closer from the mid-1940s onwards, the numbers reported in the hospital statistics for Europeans declined to single figures while Anglo-Indians were absorbed into the remaining religion and "other classes" categories.

In order to make sense of figures such as the ones above, it is important to consider changes in both nomenclature and in the wider context of social oppression; political movements and communal strife during the 1930s; the intersection of social class, caste, and religion; and shifting or fluid individual identities. Those responsible for hospital statistics were sufficiently attuned to changing socio-political preferences to move easily between and re-classify patients in the "Christian" and "other classes" categories on their books.

Gender

In contrast to caste, hospital figures for patients' gender show a more representative trend if set against gender ratios in the population overall during the 1930, when census data for both 1931 indicated equal numbers of males and females in Travancore's population.[186] This was very different from other regions in India, where males tended to consistently outnumber females on account of skewed gender preference and female infanticide amongst particular communities. Travancore hospital statistics for the 1930s, for example, mirror the census trend, being close to the 50:50 ratio, with 49 percent of men and 51 percent of women amongst patients (see Table 5.6).

Table 5.6 Attendance of in-patients and out-patients, in percentages, classified according to sexes, 1935/6 and 1945/6[187]

Sexes	1935–1936	1945–1946
Men	49%	45%
Women	51%	55%

However, subsequently a clear increase can be identified in the hospital figures between 1935/6 and 1945/6 in the proportion of women treated. This may largely be due to the fact that the Women and Children's Hospital in the capital was quite consistently listed as the institution with the highest number of in-patients and second only to the General Hospital in regard to out-patient attendance. In 1945/6 numbers in the former amounted to 14,765 (women and children) in-patients and 59,840 (women and children) out-patients. There was also a Hospital for Women and Children in Quilon. In terms of healthcare, women in Travancore were not discriminated against on account of their gender, at least not those who had local access to and were willing to embrace Western-style provision. On the basis of these figures we may conclude that in relation to general and specialist healthcare issues, gender had a bearing – at least in the capital and in provincial towns.

In this context it is worth noting that a woman, Dr Mary Poonen Lukose, became the first of her gender in the early twentieth century to be made Durbar Physician and gain a seat in the Legislative Assembly.[188] Her high social position was an important factor in her career trajectory. Mary Poonen had been "born with a silver spoon in her mouth".[189] Her family was Christian, very rich and belonged to the aristocracy. Her father, E. Poonen, held an MBBS from Aberdeen University and had been Durbar Physician and Surgeon General[190]; he was "a reputed Surgeon and a skilled physician".[191] When his daughter was appointed as a member of the Legislative Council and to a senior position in the medical service in the early 1920s, the Calcutta-based newspaper *Bengalee* noted this "very interesting news".[192] According to Raghunandan, the biographer of Maharani Setu Lakshmi Bayi (1895–1985; reigned 1924–1931), in the state the news was "received with considerable surprise".[193] But Poonen still was "accorded an enthusiastic ovation" on her first appearance in the Legislative Council. Her elevation was attributed at the time and by the Maharani's biographer to the "liberal and wise step taken by the Government of Her Highness the Maharani", rather than to Poonen's professional qualifications and influential family connections. In the 1930s, she was acting on several occasions for the European *darbar* physician, Dr James Simpson.[194] In 1938 she took over for a while from her European predecessors as Surgeon General of Travancore.[195] Apart from the apparent ease with which a woman got herself promoted to leading positions, it is important to note that from the early twentieth century onwards Western-trained Indians increasingly replaced Europeans in the medical services, mirroring similar developments in the provinces ruled by the British, where they were referred to as the 'Indianization' of the colonial services.[196] However, on account of the scarcity of women in senior positions during this period, Mary Poonen's medical appointment was as remarkable as it would have been in Britain where women fought hard to gain access to medical training and positions.[197]

Returning to the statistics discussed above, it remains to be pointed out that in contrast to general (and maternal) healthcare figures, a clear inversely gendered trend was evident in the admission registers at Travancore's mental hospital. Only 31 percent of beds were allocated to women; namely 60 of 195 in 1946.[198] This means that authorities anticipated a lower number of female patients to be present in the mental hospital. The same was the case in British-ruled provinces. However, bed capacity for women was designed to be higher in Travancore than was the case in most institutions in British India. At the Indian Mental Hospital at Ranchi, for example, on average only 20 percent of facilities were earmarked for females.[199] Contrary to expectations, bed capacity on the female wards was not reached in Travancore. For example, in 1946/7, of the total of 433 patients treated during that year, only 109 or 25 percent were women. A similar ratio prevailed in regard to admissions during the year (i.e. 49 or 20 percent of 200 new patients were female).

The religious background or "class" (as it was referred to in the reports), of newly admitted mental patients shows that the majority consisted of Hindus (67 percent), followed by Christians (29 percent), and Mohammadans (five percent) in 1946/7 (see Table 5.7).

Table 5.7 Class and sex of the patients admitted during the year 1122 [1946/7][200]

Class	Sex	Sex	Total
	Men	Women	
Hindus	105 [53%]	28 [14%]	153 [67%]
Mohammadans	9 [5%]	1 [<1%]	10 [5%]
Christians	37 [19%]	20 [10%]	57 [29%]
	151 [76%]	49 [25%]	200 [100%]

No other 'classes' were specified; that is, 'caste Hindus' were not listed separately from 'external castes' or 'other classes', as had been the case in the general health and census statistics at the time. Comparisons with other institutional and population figures are therefore difficult. However, if we are correct in assuming that the category of 'Christians' was used to designate former lower- or outcaste Hindus, it may well have been the case that caste Hindus were over-represented in the mental hospital. This would echo a similar trend in at least one institution in British India, the Ranchi Indian Mental Hospital, where a substantial proportion of inmates were drawn from the higher, but not the highest, caste communities, rather than the 'dregs of society', as is sometimes assumed. As in other statistics, the number of Muslims was more or less representative of both general and census figures (namely about 5.5 percent). However, this is also the group with the largest gender differential; only one out of ten Muslims admitted in 1946/7 was a woman (see Table 5.8).

Table 5.8 Class and sex of the patients admitted during the year 1122 [1946/7][201]

Class	Sex	Sex	Total
	Men	*Women*	
Hindus	105 [79%]	28 [21%]	153 [100%]
Mohammadans	9 [90%]	1 [10%]	10 [100%]
Christians	37 [65%]	20 [35%]	57 [100%]

Amongst Hindus and Christians, too, women were under-represented in terms of admissions, however not to the same extent as was the case in regard to Muslims.

In Travancore, Hindu and Christian women outnumbered their Muslim sisters considerably, with Hindus making up 57 percent, Christians 41 percent, and Muslims not quite 2 percent of admissions.[202] Male admissions were dominated by Hindus, who made up 70 percent, with 25 percent of Christians, and about 6 percent of Muslims. If we consider admission to a mental hospital in positive terms, we would need to judge the under-representation of women and in particular of Muslim women as an indicatation of gender discrimination or of families' disinclination to send their female relatives to a public institution. Only access to individual patient files and knowledge of the circumstances of admission and the criteria employed by certifying doctors or magistrates would allow for a sensible interpretation. Nevertheless, it can be noted that an institutional approach to mental health problems was considerably less likely to be employed in the case of women than was the case in regard to general healthcare (and, naturally, maternity services).

How then did the development of institutional mental health care, more generally, figure within the wider context of Western medical provision in Travancore?

The lunatic asylum at Trivandrum during the late nineteenth century

Provision for 'lunatics' is not discussed until the late 1860s. There is no previous correspondence regarding its necessity or of any arrangements made for the mentally ill in jails or hospital wards in earlier decades. However, during the 1860s public health more generally began to receive attention and asylums had become part of the services an aspiring modern state such as Travancore considered important. The officially recorded history of Western-style institutional provision for the mentally ill therefore starts in 1869, when a building was purchased by government "for the purpose of serving as a temporary Lunatic Asylum".[203] It was "immediately opened for the reception of the insane" in 1870.[204] The *District Gazetteer* of 1962 locates the asylum in Oolampura, a sparsely populated suburb, but Oolampura was the new site that was occupied only in 1905.[205]

The amenities were considered "very unsuitable for the treatment of the insane, yet", so the acting Dewan, V.V. Pillay noted in 1870/1, "it was the best at the time procurable".[206] He described the facilities:

> The accommodation consists of one large central hall with two good sized rooms and three small rooms on either side, all under the same roof and all more or less communicating with one another. There are good broad verandahs on all sides of the house.[207]

Judging from this description, the house may previously have been a family home and therefore not up to the ideal requirements of public asylum design then common in Western countries and in some provinces in British India. However, private institutions in Britain dedicated to the reception of higher-class, paying patients preferred buildings that resembled higher-class residencies. The homely premises in Travancore were therefore not *per se* unsuitable. As they were located across the road from the Civil Hospital, it was convenient to make use of kitchen and other facilities there, making it unnecessary to build special "cook rooms and other outhouses".[208] Despite these arrangements a number of "drawbacks" were noted that apparently made the number of reported cures effected "very fair indeed".[209] As in institutions in British India, a good proportion of the inmates consisted of violent and intractable patients, who were difficult to contain even at the best of times, let alone in the then-available building. Pillai's observations of 1870/1 echo those of so many officials in British Indian provinces at the time:

> There is at present great difficulty in disposing of the more noisy, troublesome and destructive patients. Some are at times very violent and noisy, others have strong homicidal tendencies, or strong proclivities towards arson &c. It is only by incessant watching on the part of the limited establishment attached to the new institution, that these can be prevented from doing mischief.[210]

As in British India, and in Britain itself, resources were scarce and staffing invariably limited. Plans for six padded rooms detached from the main building were recommended. This was expected to "considerably facilitate the treatment of the insane".[211] "Treatment" in this context of course referred to management, containment, and control of inmates rather than any particular medical or therapeutic measures. There was also a drive to employ those inmates who were able to do so in some kind of active pursuits and plans were afoot to engage "those trained to special work in a suitable manner".[212] Work therapy and recreational activities were common and promulgated at the time in institutions around the world.[213] The official report at Travancore did not fail to comment on the, albeit few, occupations available: "At present, the only employment which can be found for the majority of the patients is garden work, in which many of them take great interest. Every encouragement is given to their amusing themselves as much as possible."[214] Patient work in lunatic asylums was generally said to have been employed for therapeutic reasons (to provide meaningful activity), but its role in contributing to institutional finances and routine maintenance was not inconsiderable.[215]

Tabular information provided on patient numbers and disease categories was arranged on similar lines as those common in British India and Britain. During the late nineteenth and even the early twentieth centuries, mental conditions were still configured in relation to the old tripartite division of dementia, mania, and melancholia, with subdivisions for mania. Diagnostics at the time tended to rely on symptomatic behaviour and epilepsy was listed under "mania". Although the categories used in Table 5.9 seem more basic than those provided in some institutions in British India and in Britain, they were still well in line with how the insane were classified in many institutions at this period and even well into the first couple of decades of the twentieth century.[216]

Table 5.9 The following return will show the number of patients admitted, the nature of the cases treated and the results. 1870/1[217]

Disease	Remained	Admitted	Total	Discharged-cured	Discharged-relieved	Discharged-died	Remained
Dementia		13	13	7	1		5
Mania, Acut[e]		15	15	5	4	1*	5
Mania, Chronic		34	34	8	2	1**	23
Mania, Supposed		6	6	6			
Mania, Puerperalis		1	1				1
Mania, Epileptica		2	2				2
Melancholia		2	2	1			1
Total		73	3	27	7	2	37

*of Hydrothorax
**of Dysentery

Some notable features deserve comment. First, the label of 'idiocy', which was prevalent in other institutional returns, is missing here. It is of course difficult to establish if patients who would have been so designated in British Indian asylums are here subsumed under a different heading or whether intellectually disabled people were deliberately omitted from admission into the Travancore institution. There was a tendency in all asylums in India to institutionalize only the dangerous and violent; this may have had a bearing here too. In fact, the Lunacy Regulation of 1904/5 made provision only for "dangerous lunatics"; the number of private patients tended to be limited. Second, the total number of inmates admitted into the newly opened facility during its first year sounds quite considerable, amounting to 73 patients. It is likely that at least a proportion of them were previously accommodated in other places, such as the jail or hospital. The number of people confined in lunatic asylums does of course not tell us anything about the incidence of mental illness in Travancore's wider population. The great majority of people affected by mental conditions were looked after by their families, left to fend for themselves, or perhaps admitted to another public institution, such as hospital or a jail. Institutional data are only representative of the extent of institutionalization and not of the incidence of a condition amongst the wider population. Although institutional provision was very limited, and to be made available only for the violent and dangerous, authorities still tended to criticize relatives for their alleged cruelty and perceived role in making patients' conditions worse as well as their disinclination to have their family members taken to an institution. Dewan Peishkar, V.V. Pillay pondered:

> It was something even to get the patients away from the control and unkindness and even brutality of their relatives. Many of the insane of this country are rendered permanently so, I am persuaded, by the injudiciousness and even cruelty of their relatives.[218]

Pillay clearly subscribed to the idea that family care was inferior to institutional provision and that the modern ways of treating the mentally ill were preferable to traditional methods. He commented on the latter:

> On first showing any aberration of mind, they [mentally ill people] are generally supposed to be possessed of a devil and are submitted to the operations of the devil dancer, involving every kind of mental and bodily disturbance to the patient at the time when he should, above all things, be kept in quietude as far as possible, both of body and mind.[219]

Devil dancing was reviled by Europeans, especially missionaries, and high-caste Indians alike. It was practised by outcaste groups, such as the Ezhavas, who were excluded from worshipping in temples and thus followed practices considered by caste Indians as "polluting" (totem worship, demonology, animal sacrifice). As Chandramohan has shown, later caste associations such as the Sri Narayana Dharma Paripalan (SNDP), founded in 1895 by the religious reformer Sri Narayana Guru, attempted to get Ezhavas communities to engage in "Brahmanical idol worship" in new temples rather than continue with their established practices.[220] In the 1860s and 1870s, devil dancing was still widespread and a way of dealing with the mentally ill. Details of the practice were not explicated by Pillay, but its effects were condemned: "I need not here describe the ignorant brutalities which are practised on such occasions – it is enough to state that they are such as to have a most injurious influence on the condition of those subjected to them."[221]

But even if patients were spared demonic rituals, families were believed to handle the mentally ill roughly if not cruelly by means of beatings and forceful restraint to deal with intractable behaviour:

> And the unkind treatment of the insane is not confined to the primary stages of their disorder, but is too often continued during the whole of their illness while they reside in their own homes. They are often brought to the asylum with weals on their bodies from the blows which they have received or with excoriations on their limbs from the rough ropes with which they have been bound.[222]

While equipment and facilities for the kind of treatment of the insane favoured by Pillay were still lacking in the newly established institution, it was held that inmates were nevertheless dealt with in a humane manner:

> Although we have few of the appliances, in the building temporarily occupied as an asylum, for the most favourable treatment of the insane, we can yet make them tolerably comfortable, and can at least insure them kind and considerate treatment, and a proportion at least of that sympathy which appeals to the feelings of the insane as well as of those healthy in mind.[223]

As in British India, government officials in Travancore, too, considered confinement in the asylum as a boon for inmates, not only because of the "tolerably comfortable conditions" they experienced but also on account of their separation from the unkind home environment and adverse circumstances that were seen to worsen their condition.

It was not until 1877 that tangible steps were taken to replace the temporary building. Land was acquired at Pattucunnoo Hill from the Quilon Roman Catholic Mission for new premises. A long wrangle ensued between Bishop and Palace about compensation, lasting about five years. As no substitute land could be found, the mission finally had to accept monetary recompense.[224] The author of the *Travancore State Manual* of 1940, T.K. Velu Pillai (1882–1950), mentions that a separate asylum was opened a couple of years later, between 1878 and 1879, for the treatment of female lunatics.[225] Contemporary sources on the minutiae of conditions and treatments in the male and female asylums are not available. However, admission procedures were discussed extensively between 1879 and 1883. The *darbar* physician suggested to the Dewan in March 1880 that only the division magistrate or the *huzzoor* ought to be authorized to send lunatics to the asylum.[226] There had been cases when persons "whose insanity is not at all apparent" had been sent to the asylum by the sub-magistrate.[227] It was speculated that this was done to save "himself and his subordinates the trouble of collecting evidence regarding the history of mentally afflicted persons arrested in the Streets".[228] Similar cases occurred in British Indian provinces throughout the nineteenth and well into the twentieth century.[229] In this particular situation, issues of official standing too were at stake, as the *darbar* physician emphasized that "it is obviously undesirable that I should be involved in a correspondence with a Submagistrate."[230]

Following the *darbar* physician's complaint, the Dewan, N. Nanoo Pillay (1827–1886), directed that in future insane persons should be sent to the asylum through the magistrate.[231] However, there were several more cases in subsequent years when this procedure was not followed. Each time the matter was fully investigated, following in the best tradition of British-style civil administration. In one such case, the district magistrate's statement to the Dewan of December 1882 reveals some of the circumstances under which insane people came under official attention and how procedures were ignored:

> One evening at about half past six I was driving from office through the Chalay bazaar. I noticed some excitement in the crowds of people that passed. I stopped and, on enquiring, I learnt that it was caused by a lunatic running through the streets. I sent word to the beat constable, as he was not then present, to seize the madman and take him to the asylum. Since then I received no information in the matter, not even knowing whether the man was apprehended or not. If the man was presented to the Police Inspector, as is stated, he at least ought to have reported the circumstance to me which however was not done. Hence the omission to make the report as directed.[232]

Admission procedures, let alone those relating to certification of lunatics, were clearly not implemented according to rule for many years. Just a couple of months later another lunatic was sent directly to the asylum, this time by the district magistrate of Alleppey, who excused his failure to adhere to the correct procedure by telling the Dewan that he had been "fully engaged down at the Session Court" at the time the regulations had been forwarded and "consequently . . . did not recollect" them.[233] There is further, extended correspondence on procedures related to admission and discharge a couple of years later. Coordinating procedures amongst different grades of officials in varied localities constituted a challenge despite the fact that record keeping had been streamlined on the basis of the British Indian blueprint.

However, in British India, too, admission and discharge procedures were at times honoured in the breach, and relatives and doctors did not always agree on how long a patient should be confined in an institution. In the case of Travancore, in 1889, a member of the public repeatedly wrote to the *darbar* physician, Surgeon Major H.P. Esmonde White (1887–1897), to have his brother, Madaven Iyappan, discharged from the asylum.[234] On receiving a negative answer, namely that Iyappan was "not fit at present to be discharged from the Lunatic Asylum",[235] his brother, one Madhav Narayanen of Nellikaray Vedic College, sent a petition to the Dewan.[236] He explained that he had taken his brother, "who was labouring under lunacy" to the asylum for treatment and that he was now "cured of his lunacy".[237] He now wanted to have him home, fearing that "any unnecessary confinement in the lunatic asylum will again tell on his health".[238] While officials tended to suggest that families did more harm than good to their mentally ill relatives, Narayanen clearly thought that the opposite was the case. He was "even willing to bind himself by an agreement, if necessary, as to the personal security of the Patient as well as any public nuisance".[239]

Esmonde White, on his part, explained to the Dewan that he had tightened admission and discharge procedures. While hitherto patients were admitted "when brought by any one to the door and stating they were insane . . . and released on request of those who brought them", he now only admitted patients on "receiving a certificate of insanity from one of the government medical officers".[240] Like his predecessor, he insisted that "rules and regulations must be made and carried out", but while previously the town magistrate had the authority to send a person to be admitted in the asylum, it was now by force of a medical certificate only.[241] In line with procedures in British India and in European countries at this period, only medical expertise was acceptable in the certification and discharge process. Therefore, Esmonde White stressed, he cannot admit and discharge patients "until sufficient time has elapsed to allow of forming some opinion of their case".[242] Besides, while "always too anxious to allow out any of the inmates", he did not approve of turning the asylum into a "temporary rest house to suit the convenience of those with insane relatives while they go on a Journey".[243]

The correspondence shows not only the ongoing medicalization of admission and discharge procedures but also the extent to which perceptions of what a lunatic asylum ought to be differed considerably. While some members of the public, such as Narayanen, saw it as a place that temporarily could take off the pressures of care on the part of hard-pressed relatives, the medical officer in charge focused exclusively on the medical necessities of the case (and seemed also put out by the additional administrative hassles put on him by a patient's relative). From the point of view of the doctor, the walls of the asylum were to be less permeable than the world outside may have wished it to be. These differences in perspective were characteristic also of matters in British India and in Britain, where fears amongst members of the public existed that those admitted to an asylum would be left there interminably, on the authority of a medical profession keen to assert its power over medical and administrative procedures.[244] In Iyappan's case, the doctor eventually conceded that the patient was improving, adding that he "will be discharged as soon as ever I consider it safe to do so".[245] Esmonde White was clearly to labour the point about whose authority was to count in matters of patients' release. The Dewan's view was based on mainly legal considerations. In his previous correspondence to the *darbar* physician the Dewan, T. Rama Raw (Rao; 1831–1895) had weighed up in an apparently quite sensible and even-handed way the medical and legal evidence against the family's wishes laid before him:

> The petitioner persists in taking his brother out of the Asylum and promises to bind himself to look after him.
> The patient, I find is not lodged in the Asylum for any criminal offence nor does he appear to have been sent by the Police as being dangerous or

troublesome to the public. The petitioner states that he was merely brought there by himself as a private patient.

In these circumstances I am not sure whether we have the right to keep him longer in the Asylum, unless you are of opinion that he is dangerous to the public. The petitioner agrees to bind himself to take care of him.[246]

The Dewan had reached his balanced statement notwithstanding an explanatory note that had been appended to the ongoing case, which clarified that:

The lunatic not being sufficiently cured the Durbar Physician has no power to release him as we have expressly stated in a former letter to the Durbar Physician . . . that such cases should be reported to Government for orders.[247]

Medical and official government views were not always in harmony, so it seems. Officially, legal as well as medical authority as well as administrative procedures were to be observed to the letter. It took Rao's secretary a full three weeks to put matters in a conciliatory way to the petitioner, saying that the medical officer had "reported that the man is improving and will be discharged as soon as it may be safe to do so".[248]

Iyappan's case and its eventual resolution needs to be seen within the wider context of attempts to clarify the appropriate procedures and rules of administrative precedence and authority, not just in regard to medical but also penal establishments and other government departments. For example, prison regulations were changed in 1888 and the powers of the *darbar* physician clearly defined.[249] Formalized rules were of course important for public institutions in order to guard against mismanagement and arbitrary procedures, and were considered to ensure an enlightened administration guided by professional expertise, such as judicial and medical authority. In some cases this was tiresome, involving much red tape, which was not entirely in the interest of patients and their families, and may have irritated high-status European doctors who were vexed by non-compliance with mundane procedures and by outsiders' interference.

Issues of social status and precedence constituted a not always sufficiently concealed agenda in the correspondence about admission and discharge procedures, as when on one occasion in 1880 the *darbar* physician refused to engage in written exchanges with a mere sub-magistrate.[250] The caste system was extraordinarily oppressive in Travancore, creating much outrage and consternation amongst Europeans. However, on their part, too, a stringent hierarchy of social status and rules of precedence in regard to the different departments of government service was enforced not only in British Indian states, but also amongst Europeans in Princely India. For example, in 1895, the Revd C.F. Breay had asked to have made available to him and his wife a holiday bungalow in the pleasant hills of Ponmudi.[251] When the request was passed on to the Chief Engineer, W. Jopp, he put it in no uncertain terms that this was a preposterous idea. The bungalow was, so Jopp pointed out, defined as a "sanitarium for European Officers of His Highness's service".[252] The place had two sets of bedrooms, allowing two parties to stay there at the same time.

However they had to share a central hall. And it was the latter that irked Jopp, as this hall had to be shared for meals as well as double as a sitting room at other times. Therefore, if the Breays were present,

> for an Officer of the superior grades to find himself in such close social contact with a servant of the Government of lower social position would not only be extremely unpleasant to him but would be likely to be subversive of discipline.[253]

The preservation of social distance was clearly not the sole prerogative of Brahmins and other high-caste communities in Travancore. Revd Breay and his wife were not to enjoy the comfort of the hills during the hot season. Another petition to the Dewan made just a couple of months later, in April 1896, was similarly unsuccessful. The petitioner, Mr M. La Bouchardiere, who was to become Professor of English at H.H. the Maharaja's College,[254] pointed out that

> The use of the bungalow at Ponmudi is regulated by some peculiar Rules framed a long while ago which restrict the privilege of using it to a few people. As the intention of His Highnesses' Government in building the Bungalow is evidently to benefit Government officers I venture to hope that the old Rules will be interpreted or revised on a more liberal minded basis so as to enable a larger portion of His Highness' the Maha Rajah's officers to benefit by it than they have hitherto been able to.[255]

As previously, the Dewan felt disinclined to interfere with European social sentiments and referred the matter again to the chief engineer whose sensibilities had not changed, and, like the Breays, La Bouchardiere had to sweat it out in the plains.[256]

Institutional statistics and reports

Reports on public institutions such as the lunatic asylum did not contain much information on their inmates. This was the case also in British India and in Britain. In Travancore data collection was introduced relatively late in contrast to the British-ruled regions in South Asia. According to the gazetteer of 1906, no statistics on birth and deaths, nor on public health measures, were kept until 1893/4, when the Towns Improvement and Conservancy Regulation made this mandatory for the main towns and, a year later, for the whole state.[257] The post of sanitary commissioner was created as late as 1895, and information on sanitation and vaccination was collected regularly only some 42 years after British-ruled Madras had done so.[258] But even then the collection of statistical data as well as systematic public health measures tended to be largely focused on provincial towns and the vicinity of public works or plantations. Admittedly, vaccination had started in 1865, and attempts were made to reach rural locations.[259] The maharaja noted in regard to the duties of the superintendent of vaccination, installed in 1865/6, that he will need to "travel into the interior to supervise the several medical subordinates who are employed there, and to spread the benefits of medical aid in general, and of vaccination in particular".[260] At that time the superintendent, Dr Pulney Andy, MD, a "native of Madras who had taken a Diploma in Europe", supervised one "head vaccinator" and 27 subordinates.[261]

The state of "general sanitation and conservancy" received special attention whenever fairs and festivals were held. In 1900, there were 36 of these events, excluding the large Murajapom, an important sexennial festival in the capital.[262] It was pointed out that in rural areas, too, sanitary measures were adopted that year, with temporary latrines at Colachel being made permanent and a new one being provided at Poovar.[263] Sanitary intervention measures and activities undertaken by the five 'town improvement committees', which had been established in 1895 (in Trivandrum, Nagercoil, Quilon, Alleppey and Kottayam), became increasingly more interventionist. While earlier on emphasis had been on drainage and water conservancy, by 1900 the committees also "insisted" on the "systematic inspection of backyards of private premises in crowded centres".[264]

In contrast to the slow development of public health statistics and rural sanitary measures, "infirmities" were reported in the census from 1875 onwards, following British Indian census customs. In 1901, only 503 people, out of an overall population of about 3 million, were categorized as insane, a rate of 1.7 per 10,000, which, if set against data from other regions in South Asia, was favourable.[265] The Dewan assessed the comparative data, contending that "it is clear that there are relatively fewer number[s] of infirm persons in Travancore than other parts in India".[266] Only Baroda had lower ratios for reported insanity amongst its population (see Table 5.10).

Table 5.10 Number of 'insane' persons per 10,000 of the population, 1901[267]

Place	Males	Females
Travancore	2.0	1.4
Cochin	2.7	2.2
Mysore	2.1	1.6
Baroda	1.5	0.9
Madras Presidency [British India]	2.0	2.0

Intriguing as these numbers may seem, they tell us of course more about the extent to which officials managed to collect accurate details from the various communities. In regard to the tendency towards consistently lower rates being reported for females in Princely states, the Dewan suggested that these may be due to women's "general unwillingness to return their defects correctly, and the better opportunities they have than the males for concealing them from the Census enumerator".[268] He did not comment on how enumerators may have managed to extract such information from women in British-ruled Madras, where the reported male to female ratio of insanity was even. Still, like his fellow gazetteer officials in other states he did not shy away from further speculating about the causes for the male/female discrepancy, musing without corroborative evidence whatsoever that it "no doubt" showed the "greater immunity enjoyed by the female population".[269] This is in stark contrast to contentions in Britain, where females, so it has been argued, were considered during this period to be particularly prone to mental derangement on account of their physical peculiarities, namely their reproductive capacity. As Digby put it in relation to Western countries, women were restrained by a "biological straightjacket".[270] Explanations of gendered trends in the incidence and presentation of mental conditions are clearly open to speculations that are dependent on the wider cultural context by which they are framed.

As Table 5.11 shows, the statistics also revealed a local west/east divide, as higher rates of insanity, deafness, and leprosy were reported for seaside or "littoral and deltaic" areas, in contrast to those in the "mountainous and submontane" inland tracts.[271]

Table 5.11 Number of 'insane' persons per 10,000 of population, by sex, 1901[272]

Natural Divisions	Male	Female
Western (littoral and deltaic)	2.3	1.6
Eastern (mountainous and submontane)	1.5	1.2
Total	2.0	1.4

The divide was due to accessibility problems, as the Dewan himself pointed out. In 1895, the newly appointed sanitary commissioner, who had gained his experience in Madras, commented on the "considerable physical disadvantages" that impacted on the collection of vital statistics. Unlike in Madras, Travancore did not have "the village system of house-distribution for rural areas", but each house stood "in a more or less extensive compound of its own", with an "almost unbroken chain of houses extending from one end of the country to another".[273] This posed considerable problems, not only for census officials but also for those tasked with healthcare provision. Not surprisingly, the highest prevalence rate for insanity was found in the capital itself, namely 10.9 for men and 5.4 for women in every 10,000 of the population. This the Dewan attributed to, "of course", the presence of the lunatic asylum, which, he did not fail to note, was "conducted on the most approved modern lines".[274] The mere availability of an institution in a particular area creates its own momentum of usage, which was as much a factor in the higher incidence rates as the greater ease of data collection in urban areas.

Psychiatric provision at Trivandrum in the early twentieth century

Notwithstanding the inadequacies of vital statistics during the nineteenth century and the privileging of urban areas in health service delivery, Western-style mental health provision developed steadily within the wider context of the general expansion of medical services during the twentieth century. It compared very favourably with provinces directly ruled by the British. By 1900, 71 medical officers were employed in the Western-style medical department, including one male and one female surgeon, six assistant surgeons, five sub-assistant surgeons, 47 apothecaries of different grades (including three females) and 11 hospital assistants.[275] There were also 48 compounders, two matrons (for the maternity hospitals), 28 licensed midwives, and six sick nurses.[276] One Western-style medical practitioner was available for every 36,024 of the population and one hospital per 53,286 of the state's population.[277] If all officially government-aided institutions (both European and 'native') are taken into account, there was one institution per 26,368 of the population.[278]

These were impressive figures. Nagam Aiya compared Travancore's Western medical facilities to those of Madras in his 1906 *State Manual*, setting the by then 22 hospitals, 20 dispensaries, 12 government-aided institutions, as well as a leper and the lunatic asylum in Travancore against those in the British-ruled province of Madras, where there were 652 medical institutions in total, or one for every 224 square miles and every 60,510 inhabitants (in contrast to Travancore's one for every 125 square miles and 52,715 of the population).[279]

Intriguingly, in 1900, the number of people treated in European institutions fell by 2,793, while there was an increase of 5,487 in attendance at Vaidyasalas or Ayurvedic healthcare providers.[280] This can partly be explained by the increased level of support for the indigenous medicine sector and also by the fact that the new *darbar* physician, Major H. Thomson, IMS, had reduced costs by keeping a close eye on expenditure in European institutions.[281] There were other factors too that might have had an impact on the number of patients. For example, in 1904/5 the number treated dropped from 18,339 in the previous year to 7,970.[282] This considerable change had then been due to the government divesting the Sanitary Department of its established practice of giving general medical relief, confining it to the "legitimate duties pertaining to the department", namely attending only to cases of cholera and malarial fevers.[283]

Despite the generally favourable reports on medical developments in Travancore during the early twentieth century, some aspects of patient care were less commendable. The mortality rate in the lunatic asylum was high in 1900, as 13 of a total of 139 patients died that year, amounting to nearly 10 percent of patients. The *darbar* physician noted critically that the "health of the Asylum was remarkably good", but that "no satisfactory reason" was given for the high number of deaths.[284] The British resident, G.T. MacKenzie, too, remarked on the "unusually high death-rate in the Lunatic and Leper Asylums", but rather than suspecting manipulation of inmates' diets as he had done in the case of prisoners at Shenkotta Jail, he contended that "these two classes are not expected to have robust health".[285] Overall, he was therefore still inclined to commend the "good work done by the Medical Department".[286]

Conditions appear to have improved for asylum inmates, as five years later, in 1904/5, only six out of a total of 185 inmates were reported to have died (i.e. just 3 percent) and it was noted that, "The health of the Asylum was fairly good."[287] Prisoners too appear to have benefitted, as improvements in the health of convicts in the central prison were reported at the same time.[288] The British resident commented in his annual *Review on the Administration Report* on the "very marked" progress and on the "further improvements in buildings and in internal management and discipline" that had been effected.[289] Such improvements had their cost, not just in the field of healthcare, but also in other state departments. The "recurring deficits during recent years" were commented on by the resident, but the maharaja and his Dewan were still "heartily congratulated on the steady progress" made in carrying out "much-needed reforms".[290] Education had been supported in recent years, leading to Travancore boasting the highest rate of "population under instruction" of any other part of South Asia, British or Indian ruled, namely 6.64 percent.[291] In regard to the lunatic asylum, funds had been dedicated to the construction of the new institution at Oolampara [Ulampara], the provision of furniture, and annual repairs (Rs 481, Rs 988 and Rs 1,275 respectively).[292]

Venu Pillai noted in the *Travancore State Manual* of 1940, not without some discernible pride, that the name of the official term for the lunatic asylum had been changed in 1921 to "The Hospital for Mental Diseases".[293] This change of terminology took place in all institutions in British-administered India around the same time. Like many others before him, Venu Pillai contended that it was not a mere terminological issue, but implied and facilitated a new attitude towards the treatment of the insane:

> the idea of this institution as an asylum for patients from the adverse reactions of the world has been changed to that of a hospital for patients with recognisable disease forms which can be treated successfully or whose conditions may be ameliorated.[294]

He proceeded to specify the effect incurred on public attitudes: "this idea will evidently cause an unconscious influence on the public mind, since a brighter outlook on the fate of the mental patients is foreshadowed by the change in name."[295] Like V.V. Pillay had done, when he disapprovingly referred to devil dancing as a popular treatment for insanity in his *Travancore Administration Report* in the 1870s, Venu Pillai, too, criticized extant traditional perceptions: "A feeling of helplessness is induced by the fatal view that the origin of mental diseases is dependent on the visitation of the gods on some unfortunate section of humanity, or on some *karma*."[296] High-ranking state officials expressed their modernizing attitudes freely in their publications.

It is also from the 1920s onwards that an increasing number of medical staff was subsidized by government, or self-funded, to get further training overseas. For example, in 1929/30, Sub-Assistant Surgeon N.P. Nilacanta Pillai went to England for higher studies in medicine at his own expense.[297] In 1930/1, the government of Travancore sponsored A.S. Johnson, BA, MBBS to proceed to England to gain a diploma in psychiatry, guaranteeing his subsequent employment as assistant surgeon on Rs 150 per month on his return.[298] Johnson got his training at the Maudsley Hospital, which was during the early twentieth century one of the foremost training institutions in England. In British-ruled provinces, too, it was not unusual for authorities to send medical staff overseas for research or further study. For

Princely states such as Travancore, overseas studies were a welcome option for further studies, as medical colleges in India became less easily accessible to them and, if so, at increased cost. Prospective students experienced "great difficulty" in getting admission to Madras Medical College, where students from Indian states were charged "double the rate of fees prescribed for British Indian students".[299] In 1932 six places were reserved in the college for Travancorians; the state had to pay in advance to the Madras government the Princely sum of Rs 1,000 each.[300] This must have irked officials who were aware of the frequent donations made by the maharaja to institutions in British provinces.

Sending staff overseas harboured the risk of them extending their stay, as was the case not only with Johnson. Mr Velayudhan Nair LMS, too, did not come back immediately on completion of his course in ophthalmology.[301] When Johnson finally returned, in spring 1933, his presence was commented on in positive terms and the marginally richer annual reports on the institution may attest to a more medically focused rather than simply managerial approach to the treatment of the inmates.[302] Johnson was now referred to as a "specialist" and was "observed to do good and useful work in the care, attention and treatment of the mental patients".[303] He apparently studied their diseases "with a special eye on the effect of climate, drug, habit development and other environmental factors on the minds of patients".[304] However, what exactly he did was not revealed. In fact, Johnson's first report remained full of generalities, so that the *darbar* physician, James Simpson, could merely cagily note in his medical administration report for 1934/4 that, "Some clear inferences [on the effect of various factors on the minds of patients] have been reported to have been derived."[305]

Prior to Johnson's appointment, not much in terms of treatment had been reported either, with the exception of engagement in work activities. These were referred to from 1901 as occupation in the 'manufacturing department', where a weaver had been appointed that year to instruct and supervise patients.[306] The articles produced by the inmates were sold, resulting in a net profit of Rs 220–26–4.[307] By the 1920s, patients were still "engaged in jamcauls and towel weaving, coir rope making and gardening on the male side and mat weaving on the female side", although some recreation had been added, such as playing football "along with the hospital servants in the evening".[308] Given the dearth of treatments other than work, it seems indeed highly appropriate that authorities should have appointed a doctor specializing on mental illness. Johnson duly obliged, listing additional 'treatments'; these consisted of:

1   Dietetics treatment
2   Drug treatment
3   Occupational treatment
4   General and psychological treatment.[309]

What the above involved and how it affected patients' experiences was not revealed. However, Johnson's interventions did have some positive effect, as the number of deaths fell to a single figure for the first time during the 1930s.[310]

Lacking further detail, we can only speculate on the reasons for this. The gradual decrease of mortality numbers from 23 in 1930, to 16 in 1931, 13 in 1932 and, finally, nine in 1933, Johnson's first year at the institution, may well have been due to old and long-standing cases passing away over time.[311] Lower mortality rates had also been reported earlier on, in the late 1910s, following criticism of potential mismanagement or even negligence. Nevertheless, the number of patients discharged in 1933 also increased considerably, including 20 inmates out of a total of 191 whose symptoms apparently 'disappeared'. Four patients were discharged 'improved' and three 'not improved'; the latter, we may presume, on account of relatives' request or due to Johnson's endeavour to rid the institution of 'incurable' cases of long standing or of any that might have been improperly detained.[312]

During the first year of his duties, Johnson expressed his intention to open a section for voluntary boarders and an out-patient department. This was in line with the intention of the Mental Treatment Act that had then just been passed in Britain, in 1930, which permitted voluntary admission to and out-patient treatment at mental hospitals.[313] However, Johnson did not confirm individual patients' diagnoses, conveying merely his general impression that, "The cases accumulating in the Hospital are of the Schizophrenic Reaction Type."[314] An important change was the extension of additional general medical provision to the inmates. The "specialists attached to the General, and the Ophthalmic Hospitals and a Lady Doctor from the Women and Children's Hospital, Trivandrum" were "ordered to visit the Hospital for Mental Diseases, once a week". This had not been the case prior to 1934/5.[315] It is likely that these changes were implemented by Johnson, in line with what he had observed during his training at the Maudsley Hospital in England.[316] He effected other innovations too, such as "a Gramaphone with Records in Tamil and Malayalam, Foot-ball, Volly-ball, books, News papers, Magazines etc. [sic]" in order to "afford facilities for some pleasurable occupation to the patients . . . and to relieve the patients from the tediousness of their imprisoned life".[317]

Wider changes were afoot during the 1930s in the Medical Department, which included compulsory medical inspection of school children,[318] an increase in the number of nurses attached to hospitals,[319] the reassignment of professional duties, a greater degree of auditing of accounts, and un-announced ad hoc inspection of institutions.[320] The *darbar* physician, Dr James Simpson, was put in sole charge of the Medical Department; he was endowed with full administrative and disciplinary powers. Simpson immediately made "several surprise visits . . . to enquire into complaints received from the public against the Medical Officers in charge of the respective Institutions [at Chirayinkil, Kottaram, Nagercoil, Peermade]".[321] He observed several "defects" during his inspections, which led him to a number of suggestions. First, the expenditure under dieting charges and hospital necessaries had to be audited more closely; second, the stock of furniture, cooking utensils, and surgical instruments had to be regularly checked against the inventory and any losses had to be explained; third, menials needed to be on duty in dispensaries whenever there were any in-patients present and a duty roster had to be arranged so that patients were not left without hospital servant during the night.[322] Simpson aimed at eradicating mismanagement and negligence. He was adamant that discretion should be made "in giving diets to the really indigent persons and diet sheets sent to Office with an account of the amount expended for sanction" rather than requisitioning "uniform expenditure (for milk, sago, kerosene oil, firewood etc.) irrespective of Market fluctuations and the number of patients accommodated".[323]

Outright fraudulent practices had come to officials' notice, too. It was noted that, "the Public have a mistaken impression that medical aid can be obtained in Government Institutions only on payment of fees."[324] A notice was therefore circulated "to all the Medical Officers in charge of Medical Institutions to see that it is hung on a very conspicuous place in the institution for the information of the Public".[325] It read: "Medical and Surgical advice, treatment and medicines are free to all patients in Government Institutions. Any breach of the above rule should be reported to the Durbar Physician."[326] All was not well in the state of Travancore, but in mitigation it has to be noted that similarly deplorable abuses occurred in British-ruled states too.

Whether fees ought to be charged was debated frequently and the policy consequently changed back and forth over time. In 1939/40, "as usual", free medical aid and free supply of medicines was available in all government-maintained medical institutions.[327] In 1941/2, a levy for medicines and medical attendance was introduced. The fees collected during the following year amounted to about Rs 10,000.[328] General austerity measures introduced during the Second World War may have swayed government views towards medical charges, in particular since the invasion of Burma by the Japanese in December 1941. As part of attempts to reduce expenditure, retired physicians and surgeons were asked to help out and donations by the general public were actively solicited[329] at a time when medical personnel deployed in the Travancore State Forces were on duty in British India and medical officers were granted emergency commissions in the Indian Army Medical Corps (IAMC).[330] In 1943/4 alone, ten medical officers, including Assistant Surgeon A.S. Johnson from the mental hospital, were given leave to join the IAMC. Johnson, the trained expert in psychiatry, left the Hospital for Mental Diseases in the hands of a generalist just ten years after his appointment.

The years since Johnson's arrival in 1933 were characterized by frequent staff in managerial changes in the mental hospital and in other medical departments. For example, during his leave of absence in 1936/7, an officer from the "General cadres" was put in charge" for about three and a half months.[331] More encouragingly, a year later, in 1937/8, a "Lady with LMP Diploma was appointed as Matron on Rs 40 per mensem" to look after the women in the female section.[332] (The LMP or Licentiate in Medical Practice was a qualification specific to British colonies and consisted of a five-year course, with a narrower curriculum than the British MBBS.) Despite, or rather because of, the detrimental impact of the Second World War on conditions in British India and, by proxy, in Indian states, and the continued movement of staff it brought with it, a number of changes were made in the medical department. For example, classes were started for the training of compounders, midwives and *dhais* [traditional Indian midwives] (with 23, 40 and 21 pupils respectively) to compensate for shortfalls in medical provision;

these were facilitated by continued donations from the public.[333] Yet, it was not until 1946/7 that nurses were employed in the mental hospital; two male "other nurses" are referred to in the official reports.[334] During this period, the decentralization of administration known in Travancore as the "District Medical Scheme" was implemented.[335] This followed similar arrangements made in British India in 1919, where it was referred to as the "provincialisation" of government services. However, the mental hospital in the capital remained under the direct control of the surgeon general and in Johnson's absence during the war, Mr V. Kumara Pillai made deputy surgeon in charge; Kumary Pillai had no specialist training in psychiatry, but was well qualified as a generalist.[336]

Pillai continued at the mental hospital until 1947, when he was sent to America to enhance his professional expertise.[337] Other medical doctors too were lined up to get further qualifications abroad, and the United States were a preferred location.[338] However, it had proved difficult to get "admission for foreign Doctors for advance studies in the Universities and Medical Schools in the U.S.A." and it was therefore decided that

> Messrs Jacob Taliat and V. Kumara Pillai, candidates selected from the Medical Department for higher technical training need not undergo any academic course but that it would be enough if they visit the important Medical Institutions in the U.S.A. and U.K. to acquaint themselves with the new developments in medicine and surgery and contact eminent members of the profession.[339]

This was well in line with what was happening in other Princely states and British-ruled provinces.[340] Britain was no longer the main destination of choice considered by the Indian elite for training in the modern methods of medicine. The British *Raj* had come to an end; it had also long ceased to be the exclusive fountain of all modern wisdom and expertise for elite groups in South Asia.

Formal classification and treatment of patients

The classification scheme used at the mental hospital from at least 1944/5 if not the early 1930s onwards, was based on the one introduced by the Swiss-American Adolf Meyer (1866–1950) in the United States in the early part of the twentieth century.[341] It was then brought to England and Scotland by British disciples who had trained under him at the Phipps Psychiatric Clinic at Baltimore where Meyer had become director in 1908. Upon returning to Great Britain, psychiatrists such as D. K. Henderson (1884–1965) in Scotland, and Australia-born Aubrey Lewis (1900–1975) and Glaswegian R. D. Gillespie (1897–1945) in England had become leading academics in their own right and taught Meyerian psychiatry.[342] Hence psychiatrists from India training in Great Britain during the interbellum period or in some places in the United States were influenced by Meyer's classification. Johnson received his specialist training in psychiatry at the Maudsley Hospital and seems to have introduced Meyer's classifications to Travancore. In Meyer's terminology, "reaction", as used in the classification in Table 5.12, had a

Table 5.12 Types of mental diseases in the mental hospital during the year 1120 [1944/5][343]

I. Affection Reaction Types
  1. Manic Depressive Psychosis
      a. Hypomania
      b. Acute Mania
      c. Delerious mania
      d. Simple Retardation
      e. Acute Depression
      f. Depressive Stupor
      g. Chronic Mania
      h. Alternating States
      i. Mixed States
  2. Involutional Melancholia
II. Schizophrenia Reaction Types
    a) Simplex
    b) Hebephrenia
    c) Katatonia
    d) Paranoid States
III. Paranoia, Paranoid Reaction Types
  1. Paraphrenia
  2. Paranoia
      a) Eccentric
      b) Egocentric
IV. Organic Reaction Types
  1. General Paralysis of the insane
  2. Tabes with Psychosis
  3. 3. Disseminated Sclerosis with Psychosis
  4. Epidemic Encephalitia with Psychosis
  5. Psychosis of Senility
      i. Arteric sclerosis
      ii. Presbyophrenis
      iii. Alzheimer's Disease
  6. Cerebral Tumour
  7. Traumatic Psychosis
  8. Thyroid Disease with Psychosis
  9. Other Endocrine disease with Psychosis
  10. Other diseases with Psychosis
V. Toxic Psychosis
    A. End[e]genous group drug addictions
      1. Alcoholic Psychosis
      2. Opium Habit
      3. Ganja habit

B. Exogenous Group
   Acute confusional Insanity
C. Endogenous group following
   1. Nephritis
   2. Diabetis
   3. Reproduction
   4. Cardic Vascular Diseases
   5. Other Diseases
VI. Epilepsy & Epileptic Equivalents
   A. Epilepsy
   B. Equivalents
      1. Tran[c]ient
      2. Protracted Delirium
   C. Epileptic Dementia
VII. Psyc[h]o Neurosis
      1. Hysteria
      2. Anxiety Neurosis
      3. Obsessional Neurosis
      4. Neurasthenia
VIII. Mental Defect
IX. Perversions of Sex Instincts
X. Under Observation

---

technical meaning and was meant to highlight that all psychiatric disorders were only biological "responses" or "reactions" to psychosocial *noxa* or something that exerts a harmful effect on the body.

In terms of diagnostic nomenclature, the mental hospital at Trivandrum was from the 1930s onwards well up to date with what was done at some of the most prominent research institutions in Britain and the United States. To what extent this helped diversify and improve the treatment of inmates, leading to better patient experiences, is difficult to ascertain. Some of the treatments discussed in the annual reports were clearly in line with those applied overseas. For example, an electroshock apparatus was installed in 1944/5 and V.K. Pillai, who was then in charge, was "deputed to Madras to get himself acquainted with the working of the apparatus".[344] Apparently, the apparatus was subsequently "operated successfully and many patients" were reported to have "benefited by the same".[345]

In 1944/5, a total of 323 men and 109 women were treated in the hospital. As Table 5.13 indicates, the percentage of females undergoing electrotherapy was therefore higher than male treatment rates, namely 46 percent for the former and 28 percent for latter. About a third of inmates benefitted – or suffered, as the case may be – from it. If we are inclined to see electrotherapy as a positive approach, we would consider females to have benefitted from it disproportionately. However, we

Table 5.13 Therapy work in the Travancore Mental Hospital: electrical, by sex and outcome, 1946/7[346]

	Treated	Cured	Improved	Not improved	Remaining
Males	90	40	23	8	19
Females	50	18	14	6	12
Total	140	58	37	14	31

do not know the criteria employed in the selection of candidates considered suitable for this treatment and hence it is difficult to interpret female predominance in the above figures. Similar problems apply to the percentage of women considered "cured" following the application of the procedure; it was lower than that of men (namely 36 percent and 44 percent respectively), while a roughly equal percentage of female and male patients were described as "improved" (28 percent and 26 percent respectively).

The gendered treatment pattern was reversed in the case of light therapy (see Table 5.14). In this case, men were more likely to be selected (i.e. 17 percent of males, in contrast to 6 percent of females). Alas, the same reservations as prevail in regard to electrotherapy. We can only speculate that the treatments entailed 'photo' or 'light therapy', which was popular from the late nineteenth century onwards, when Niels Finsen (1860–1904) had employed it mostly in cases of lupus and skin disorders.[347] It was also considered to have a soothing effect.

Table 5.14 Therapy work in the Travancore Mental Hospital: light treatment, by sex, 1946/7[348]

	Males	Females	Children	Total
Ultra-violet	26	5	1	32
Infrared	9	2	–	11
Total	35	7	1	43

As in earlier periods, patients continued to be employed in various "occupational industries", such as the "1. Manufacture of Jamackals and towels, 2. Coir making, and 3. Gardening for the males and mats making for the females".[349] "Amusement" remained restricted, if compared to other institutions,[350] consisting merely of "a Gramaphone and a radio set", while "those who could read [were] supplied with illustrated papers, news papers, novels and Malayalam periodicals".[351]

Institutional trends and statistics

As can be seen from Figure 5.2, the number of patients passing through the lunatic asylum increased slowly from the date of its inauguration in 1870/1 until a couple of years before British India's Independence and Travancore's short-lived independence as a country separate from the Indian Union. This trend was followed by a sharp rise of numbers in 1946/7.[352]

Figure 5.2 Number of patients present at beginning of year; admitted, discharged, and died during the year; total treated and remaining at the end of the year, between 1870/1 and 1946/7[353]

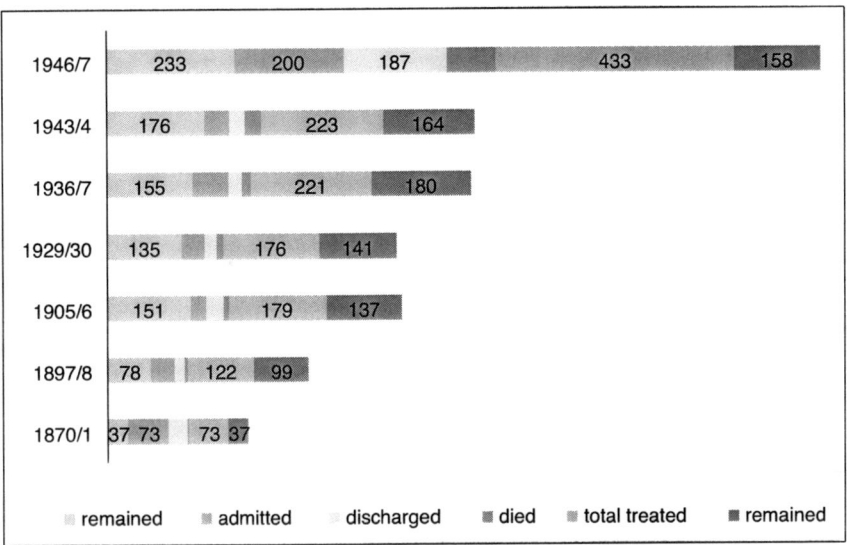

In 1946/7, the number of patients admitted increased by a factor of three to four in contrast to earlier years; discharges were six to ten times higher; deaths three to 44 times higher and numbers treated two to six times higher. What drove these changes towards the end of the Princely era is not commented on in the annual reports. The most plausible suggestion would be that the figures for 1946/7 included both in- and out-patients; yet, the reports refer consistently to in-patients only. Whatever may have been the case, the work atmosphere for staff and the experience of patients would have changed dramatically in 1946, as a much larger number of patients as had hitherto been the case was being processed and seen, alive or dead, by staff. The resources required to do so would have been considerable, even if high turnover rates of patients, as indicated by the raised number of discharges (and deaths!), are taken into account. It is likely that conditions deteriorated considerably. The period when inmates became inhabitants of "dens" and the institution "an unruly prison and torture centre" may have had its beginnings at that point.[354]

The phenomenon of high death rates amongst mental hospital patients during periods of war is of course well documented. Some of the most serious evidence has been provided by von Bueltzingloewen who showed that some 40,000 to 45,000 patients starved, or rather were left to starve, to death during the Nazi occupation of France (1940–1945).[355] The population of Travancore was of course not directly occupied by a foreign power, but here too austerity measures and staff shortages in medical institutions affected patients. As Figure 5.3 shows, the percentage of patients shot up from single figures, hovering around six to seven percent during the first three decades of the twentieth century, to double figures and two and even three times the previous ratio, in 1943/4 and 1946/7, respectively. But previously also high death rates during particular years.

Figure 5.3 Percentage of patients who died, of total number treated during the year, 1870–1947[356]

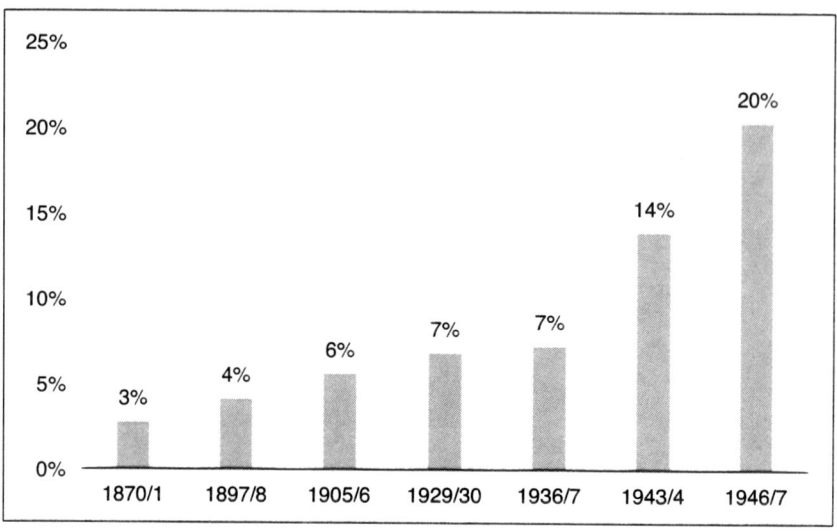

The steadily increasing mortality rate from 1870 to the first decade of the twentieth century documents a similarly bleak process, as it doubled over this period. It would of course be wrong to conclude that modern psychiatry as extant during the early part of the twentieth century was to blame for this trend. Many other factors are implicated in reported death rates, such as the admission policies prevalent at different periods, the health status of patients prior to admission, general conditions in the institution, and the percentage of old and long-term patients amongst inmates. If taken at their face value, the above figures compare well with those reported for lunatic asylums in British-ruled India during the late nineteenth century. They are also in line with the figures at the majority of mental hospitals there in the twentieth century.[357] As many institutions in British India did not keep records regularly during the Second World War, or limited inpatient facilities, it is difficult to tell if Travancore was out of step with what was happening in other regions during this period. It was definitely not in keeping with the percentage of mortality in all other medical institutions in the state, which amounted to 2.43 percent in 1946/7.[358]

It is clear though from the data that the institutional policy at the Trivandrum Mental Hospital had changed during the War. There was an ambition to keep the number of inmates staying at the institution as low as possible, despite highly increased admission figures.[359] Figure 5.4 shows that the ratio of patients remaining at the close of every year was the lowest by far in 1946/7 of any year before.

Figure 5.4 Percentage of patients remaining at the end of the year, of total number treated, 1870–1947[360]

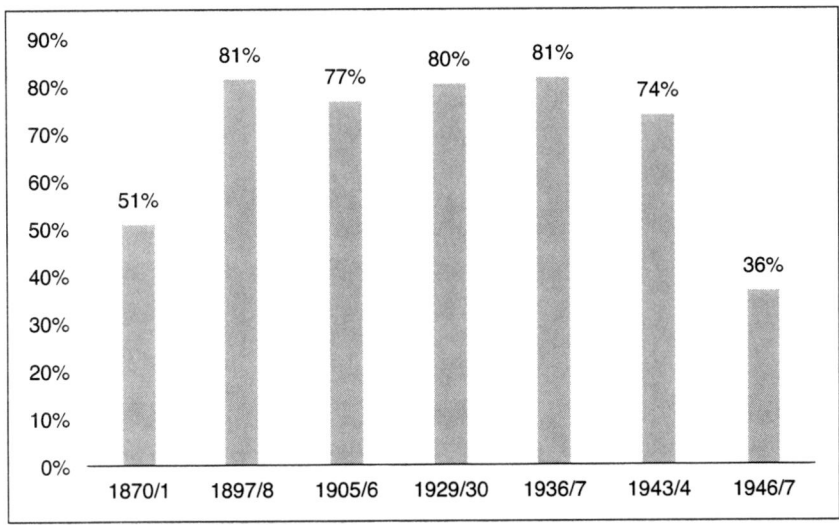

Only a little more than one-third of patients treated in 1946/7 remained in the institution. The aim may well have been to keep the number of chronically ill or "incurable" patients low; this kind of patient tended to accumulate in mental institutions over time. The consistently high rates reported for all other years, except when the asylum was opened, may indicate that the majority of inmates at Travancore were made up of long-standing cases, like in Britain, where institutions began to 'silt up', as it was then referred to, with the chronically ill, just a couple of decades after the mandatory opening of public institutions following the County Asylums Act of 1845. Figure 5.5, showing the percentage of patients discharged, seems to support this suggestion in regard to what was happening in 1946/7.[361]

Figures for 1870/1 are unusual, as this was the year when the first batch of patients were received in the newly opened premises. Assessment at the asylum of people presented for admission is likely to have led to a considerable number to be considered unsuited for continued care at buildings that, as we have seen, were not properly set up for the confinement of certain groups, such as violent inmates. In contrast, the sheer number of patients sent to the hospital in 1946/7 would have encouraged high discharge rates.

The impression that can be gleaned from the annual reports is one of doctors' and administrators' awareness of what is needed in a mental hospital to ensure its smooth running. As far as admission procedures, record keeping, and attention to statistical trends such as mortality rates were concerned, these compared well with those in British India and overseas. However, unlike in reports from other medical institutions in Travancore, and in comparison to mental hospitals such as in Princely Mysore and Ranchi in British India, no particularly energetic

Figure 5.5 Percentage of patients discharged, of total number treated during the year, 1870–1947

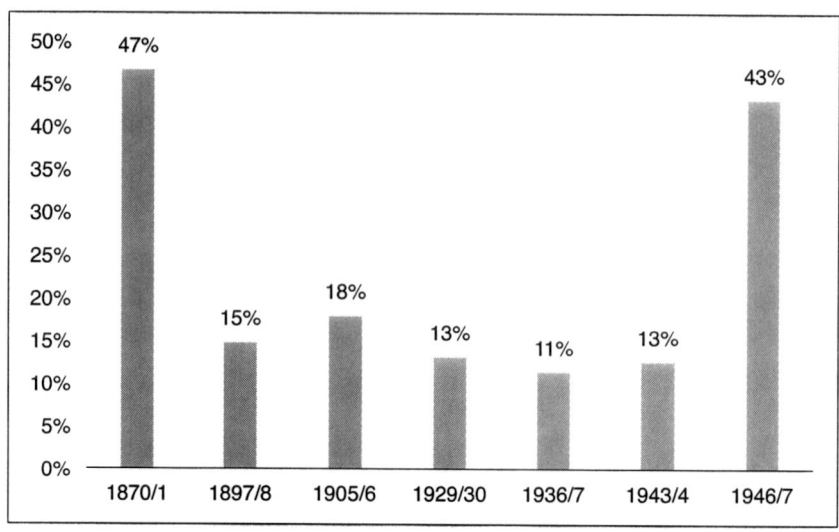

engagement with the specifics of medical treatment can be identified. Emphasis is on managerial basics such as work, minor recreational pursuits, and attention to diet. The scope for medical intervention was of course generally restricted in regard to mental illness until the 1920s, when new approaches – however cruel and outlandish they may appear to present-day observers – were trialled in many institutions across the globe. Johnson broke the mould to a certain extent during the late 1930s, but his more psychiatrically-focused regime seems to have vanished once he left the hospital after six years and was replaced by his non-psychiatrically trained successor.

It would have been a challenge for Johnson to implement the kind of approach he had become familiar with during his training at the Maudsley. It would not have helped that he did not get any encouragement in his attempts from the Maudsley's director, Edward Mapother. In his unofficial review of mental health provision in India of 1938, Mapother commented on conditions in Trivandrum. He had not visited Travancore during his India tour, but Johnson sent him a lengthy report.[362] Reflecting on the material, Mapother mused that Travancore was "in some respects one of the most progressive States in India".[363] In particular, he referred to the level of literacy, which was then the highest of all British and Indian states. However, he was not, as he put it, "greatly impressed by the very long Annual Report" that he had received.[364]

Mapother had very clear ideas about how a modern psychiatric institution ought to be run. He frequently criticized even colleagues in Britain who held different views to him or found themselves struggling in woefully under-funded county mental hospitals crowded with 'chronic cases'; he managed to antagonize many of them. His 'model' institution was his own Maudsley Hospital, run as a research-based facility along the lines of establishments in continental Europe, such as in Munich. The Travancore Mental Hospital in the 1930s, albeit located in a 'model state', did not meet the standards he expected. Even in relation to most institutions in British India, except at Madras and Ranchi (at the European Mental Hospital) his judgement was harsh. Only the mental hospital in Princely Mysore met his criteria and standards fully to the extent that he considered it as "almost unique among mental Hospitals in India".[365] As far as the 'model' state of Travancore was concerned, not all of its medical institutions were located at the cutting edge of institutional provision, at least not in the view of research-focused clinicians such as Mapother. In this respect Travancore was not unusual if compared to most of the psychiatric facilities available in British India and in Britain itself. In some regions, such as the Orissan Princely states, no state-sponsored mental health provision existed.

The Orissan states – "something rotten somewhere"

The journalist and editor of the Delhi-based newspaper *Current Affairs*, S.P. Sharma, affirmed in 1942 that "The Oriya [Orissan] has perhaps been amongst the most unfortunate persons in modern India."[366] Major problems were in his view floods, famines, and cyclones; the fact that nearly two-thirds of the population were aboriginals and hence "undeveloped"; communications were inadequate and affected commerce detrimentally; and people had to "stint and starve" to "satisfy the demands of an effete and unconscionable zamindari system", while the region was blessed with vast yet undeveloped resources.[367] Sharma applied this description to British Orissa, namely the areas ruled directly by the colonial power. He considered the situation in the 26 Orissan states ruled by local princes just as bad, with the additional problems incurred by what he referred to as "grave misrule".[368] Sharma investigated further and concluded that there was "something rotten somewhere".[369]

As Mishra, Pati, and others have shown, there was indeed something very rotten in the Orissan states.[370] The majority of the population was heavily exploited over the centuries, being subject to oppressive land tenure systems, heavy taxes and practices such as *rasad, magan, and bethi*.[371] Following the cynical logic of exploitation, *bethi* or forced unpaid labour could be justified on account of people's abject poverty, making them unable to pay taxes.[372] *Rasad* or free hospitality had to be accorded to visiting officials, and *magan* or presents to rulers were expected on occasion of Hindu festivities and royal and other dignitaries' family celebrations. The "normal" working day might be 11 hours, as in the case of Kalahandi, which was honoured by the British with a nine-gun salute from the late nineteenth century onwards.[373] Pati characterizes the varied systems of land tenure and levies as a "co-existence of monetization and feudal exploitation, which crippled the people", systems that were largely designed or introduced by the British by means of permanent revenue settlement, while the preservation of existing practices of syphoning off the major part of any surplus of agricultural production was condoned.[374]

Political movements and uprisings from the late nineteenth century onwards expressed people's dissatisfaction. During the most widespread, the so-called prajamandal demonstrations, in the wake of the Orissa States Peoples Conference of 1937, the colonial authorities in the British-ruled areas lent, as Sharma put it, "the full weight of its physical force to the troubled Rulers to restore order within their territories".[375] The quelling of unrest by the British was nothing new. As long as internal peace and order was maintained, the British were more or less indifferent to what was happening to the people at the hands of princes as long as the supreme power received its annual *peshkush* or levy and was guaranteed access to natural resources such as Talcher's coal and Mayurbhanj's timber and iron ore. The growing strength of the prajamandal movement, however, demanded particularly swift and "vexatious interference".[376] After all, this movement directly challenged both Princely and colonial rule.

Importantly, while Princely rule in some of the Orissan states may largely have been portrayed by the British as 'backward' and 'despotic', they profited at the same time economically from the very features, which were the hallmarks of this backwardness and despotism: oppression and exploitation. Throughout the period of British supremacy, formal intervention in Princely internal affairs was considered only once rioters were seen to be a potential threat to economic profitability and political stability in the wider region, and hence to colonial rule itself. As W.W. Hunter put it in hegemonically sanitized but no uncertain terms in his *Statistical Account of Bengal* of 1877:

> Hid away in these natural vastnesses, the aboriginal tribes continue to enjoy the freedom which they love, under the nominal rule of hereditary Hindu chiefs. The Paramount British Power rarely interferes; but it is promptly felt wherever anarchy or outrage has to be repressed, or commerce encouraged.[377]

The rhetoric of the civilizing mission and of modernity that went hand in glove with policy guidance on welfare policies and administrative reforms in states such as Travancore and Mysore became prominent in the Orissan states only once the actual threat of people's movements came to outweigh the convenience and profitability of complacent non-interference in existing systems of surplus extraction. Concern about Indian people's welfare was not universally prevalent nor translated into any remedial policy measures, but was dependent on the ease with which regional power in British and Princely-ruled Orissa could be maintained. Indirect colonial rule came in many shapes and forms, and medicine and health services were not always and necessarily part of the process of modernization encouraged by the supreme power.

Princely rule, too, came in many shapes and forms in the over 20 or so Orissan states that covered about 30,000 square miles, with a population of 50 million in the 1930s. Individual states ranged in size from about 4,000 square miles and a population of nearly 1 million (Mayurbhanj) to only 46 square miles and just 25,000 inhabitants (Tigiria).[378] On account of the high percentage of tribal peoples such as the Santhals and Kols, they were invariably considered by the British and by most (settled) Indians alike as 'primitive' and 'backward'. Being semi-nomadic and organized in tribes constituted a challenge to the boundaries of geographic localization that was necessary for predictable and easy revenue collection, in British-ruled areas as much as in those under Princely governance. At the same time it made it easier to subjugate them militarily – at least temporarily. The British gained paramountcy over most states during the decades following the defeat of the Marathas in 1803, and subsidiary alliances were subsequently entered into with local princes. The subordinate states were first an additional duty of the commissioner of the British-ruled Orissan states in Cuttack; then controlled by a political agent based at British-held Sambalpore; and when the new province of Bihar and (British-ruled) Orissa was formed in 1912, these "feudatory states of Orissa" were overseen by the government based in Patna. From 1935, when British Bihar and Orissa were split, they came again under the purview of a political agent based in Sambalpur.

So, how did mental health care figure in the various states? Given that exploitation levels in the Orissan states were so woefully high and a large proportion of the populace scarcely managed to scrape a living, it would be naïve to expect anything much in terms of support for the mentally ill. A comparatively small number of subjects that consisted predominantly of subsistence-farming, semi-nomadic tribal communities had to produce both the annual "subsidy" to the British and the means to maintain the local aristocracy and its toadies. As has been shown, even in the best of states, such as Travancore, social welfare and medical measures for the majority of people outside urban centres were not a high priority, unless particular problems such as famines, plague, smallpox, malaria, and cholera affected commerce or threatened urban communities. There were no big cities in the Orissan states until later in the twentieth century. In the 1870s, for example, "not a single city" existed and there were "only six villages of more than five hundred houses, and only two of more than a thousand".[379] Given the absence of urban centres and of a vocal elite that subscribed to Western ideas of economic and moral uplift of the masses rather than economic and cultural self-aggrandisement, bricks and mortar manifestations of modernization along Western lines such as hospitals and schools were therefore less likely to emerge.

In his *Orissa, or the Vicissitudes of an Indian Province under Native and British Rule*, Hunter had observed in 1872 that even in British-ruled Cuttack district "the Civil Surgeon, after five years' residence in the District, reports that he has not observed any improvement in the health of the inhabitants during this period."[380] This, he argued, was largely due to people's ignorance, as was illustrated in regard to their response to smallpox: "it is no uncommon sight to see people in the streets, or walking about the crowded market-places, covered with the disease."[381] He concluded that, "Ancient prejudice stands in the way of vaccination."[382] Legitimation of rule was achieved by means of religion, appeal to royals' ancient lineages that established a link with tribal ancestry, as well as forced dispossession of land and brutal oppression. As Pati has shown, the Hindu princes gained legitimacy by means of integrating certain Adivasi cults into the Hindu pantheon. Tribals' loyalty was strengthened by, as Pati puts it, "rulers' encouragement and support of *adibasi* traditions and customs", such as the annual *ratha jatras*, connected with the famous Puri Jagannatha or chariot festival.[383] Even tribal healing rituals became Hinduized and incorporated into Princely ceremonies. Pati gives the example of the tribal deification of trees and plants and the royal courts' incorporation of associated worship practices, such as the *bhramaramari* worship,[384] into a regular procedural by means of court-appointed tribal priests or *dehuri*, who thereby became empowered by the rulers to lead the sacred ceremonies, and their villages received royal patronage while they were simultaneously being incorporated into the web of royal power.[385]

Within this order of legitimacy, appeals to modern, enlightened policies and the civilizing mission were still possible, but not pressingly necessary. Modern medicine and its institutional trappings did not figure to any great extent in the arsenal of Princely internal policies. Mental health, which was not high on the list of priorities even in states most vociferously devoted to the project of a Western-framed modernity, was unlikely to gain a prominent role in the Orissan states. Apart from hagiographers concerned with trumpeting the supposedly just rule and the fantastic riches accumulated by royal lineages, historians of Orissa agree that the people and particularly the tribals suffered woefully from the double yoke of British and Princely rule. British officials were at times ruthless and wilfully ignored appeals for the need to "uplift" backward tribals and poor castes and outcastes. In fact, tribal people or Adivasi were subject to mockery and denigration on the part of both Europeans and non-tribal Indians. Hunter noted that,

> During many centuries Orissa stood forth not only as the most orthodox, but also as the most ignorant, of the Hindu Provinces of India. 'As stupid as an Uriya' became a proverb with the . . . inhabitants of the adjoining Gangetic delta. A more elaborate aphorism declares: 'The people of the extreme east of Bengal are not men, but the Uriya is a beast. He climbs trees and jumps like a monkey, though he has no tail.[386]

And as is well known from the history of slavery and racism, those who are likened to beasts and monkeys are not accorded the respect and human values considered applicable to those who see themselves superior to them. Adivasis were located at the bottom of the imperial and Princely pecking order.[387]

Despite the backwardness attributed to people in Orissa by Europeans and Indians in other provinces, some states were still considered as 'model states'. Dhenkanal, famous for its timber production and tigers, was considered by the British as a principality that was retrieved from a "miserable state" marred by "family feuds and follies" to a well-managed state during the latter part of the nineteenth century.[388] Its ruler even received the title of *Maha*raja from the British "as a reward for the moderation and justice" with which he was seen to rule his people and following the "charity" he showed in the wake of the famine of 1886.[389] Such honours made no allusion to the existence of forced labour and other oppressive practices.

Nor did they prevent contemporary observers such as Hunter from ridiculing the ruler's tastes, intellectual abilities, and policies, when he noted that during a visit he was "called in to admire a curious medley of the costliest objects of art mingled with the pettiest gimcracks".[390] However, Hunter did commend the maharaja doing "justice in public sessions to his people" and for keeping "his prisoners hard at work upon the roads".[391]

In an anecdote titled "Jail System in a Model State", Hunter commented on the jail that consisted of two sheds, one of which was "monopolized by ten men, whose light complexion declared them to belong to the trading class", while in the other were crowded 59 men.[392] While the former "lolled at great ease and in good clothes in their prison-house", the latter were "packed as closely as sardines, and with no other clothing except a narrow strip round their waist".[393] When quizzed on the situation by Hunter, the maharaja was recorded as saying: "But then the ten are respectable men, and of good caste, while the fifty-nine are mere wood-men [Adivasi]; and it is only proper to maintain God's distinction of caste."[394] Given that His Royal Highness was known to have displayed a "courteous and intelligent demeanour" and to "suit his conversation to the supposed taste of the British Officer", any joke or censure relating to the situation portrayed by Hunter would have been on the British as well as the Indian side.[395] After all, as has been shown, British colonial jails were not altogether known for their salubriousness and humanity either and an argument of social distinction and segregation by class invariably appealed to the class-conscious British.[396]

Unlike most other Orissan states, Dhenkanal had a school and a charitable dispensary. Both were framed, according to Hunter's dubious sardonic sense of humour, "on the model of our own [i.e. British-run] Bengal institutions of the same sort, especially in the number of registers kept, and the multitudinous returns regarding the pupils and patients".[397] The joke would have been equally valid had a lunatic asylum existed in Dhenkanal or in any of the other Indian states. Model Indian princes such as the ruler of Dhenkanal followed British practices to the letter when they intended to please the power that kept them on the *gadi*. Any health measures provided on the basis of this blueprint were as hollow in British-ruled Bengal and in Dhenkanal as, in the view of some historians and ethnographers, the crowns that Princely rulers were endowed with by the British.[398]

Still, despite his aloof mockery, Hunter and his contemporaries during the late nineteenth century considered Dhenkanal as "the most civilized" of the Orissan Princely states. In the field of health services it could boast at least a dispensary of sorts. Meanwhile, people's concerns, as expressed during the demonstrations of 1938, related to continued ruthless deforestation and violation of excise laws. Nanda reports that 60,000 peasants from Dhenkanal marched to Cuttack.[399] Their demands included civil liberties and responsible government, abolition of *bethi* and *magan*, export–import restrictions, and enforcement of tenancy and forest laws.[400] The necessities of survival they focused on concerned economics, labour conditions, and political representation, not health provision and social welfare.

Although the prajamandal and other peasant movements were less significant in Mayurbanj in the 1930s (sometimes referred to as Morabhanj), oppression and exploitation were rife there too. Its ruler was accorded the title of *Maharaja* on account of his successful defeat of an uprising during the Indian Revolt of 1857.[401] Its history was no less turbulent than that of most other states. According to Hunter, the British realized in the very early nineteenth century that if they "were to live in peace with the hill chiefs", they would need to "tax them very lightly".[402] However, once the state was under Princely rule, the tribute to the British was a mere £106 per annum, while the raja's official income amounted to an enormous £10,000, "but probably very much more".[403] Rebellion, according to Hunter himself "brought on by the oppression of the aboriginal population by the petty officials of the Raja", was rife and was quelled only with the help of the British.[404] Apologetically, Hunter was quick to affirm that the population's situation had been even worse under the Marathas, who had conquered the region prior to their defeat by the British.[405]

Like other British administrators, Hunter was keen to portray Mayurbhanj as a well-run state. The idea that, unlike most of the other Orissan states, Mayurbhanj was 'progressive' has endured well into the post-colonial period. D.M. Praharaj, for example, described it as recently as 1988 as "an excellent example of benevolent administration under the Rajas and their enlightened bureaucrats".[406] He even suggested that, "The society of Mayurbhanj is an ideal synthesis of tribal and non-tribal elements due to the co-existence of these two major groups of people."[407] How authors such as Praharaj manage to reconcile these statements with evidence of exploitation, continued uprisings, and people's movements beggars belief.

The tribal element of Mayurbhanj society was described in varied ways in the earlier literature. Hunter proclaimed that: "The inhabitants of this wild region form one of the ethnical curiosities of the world."[408] Alongside this, the Romantic trope of the noble savage prevailed, as in a report by Major S.C. Macpherson, in which the "character" of "the Kandh race" [Khond] was summed up in reference to favoured nineteenth-century traits:

> A passion to love of liberty, devotion to chiefs, and unconquerable resolution. They are, besides, faithful to friends, brave, hospitable, and laborious. Their vices, on the other hand, are the indulgence of revenge, and occasionally of brutal passion; Drunkenness is universal; the habit of plunder exists in one or two small Districts alone.[409]

In some nationalist accounts soon after Indian Independence, and in contrast to Praharaj, writers such as S.C. Bose, member of the Orissa Chamber of Commerce and the Indian Council of Foreign Trade, portrayed Adivasis's characteristics sympathetically, commenting on their degradation on account of unsympathetic policies:

> Being savage in environment and illiterate regarding education th[is] mobile mass of human force is thrown out from place to place in search of employment and at last they are exploited to the maximum by the accumulated few. They have a great culture, probably higher than that of the Aryans. . . . But the recent turn of tide has made them 'Coolies'.[410]

Yet, despite Orissa-wide oppression, Mayurbhanj, like Dhenkanal, could boast at least some education and health measures, introduced in the 1870s, for which the then-ruler Krishna Chandra Bhanj was created Maharaja in 1877. His administration was considered by the British as "efficient" and his "public liberality" was praised, in particular the donation of Rs 27,000 towards Cuttack High School (later Ravenshaw College) – in *British*-ruled Orissa![411] The fact that he had been "assisted and advised" when he assumed the *gadi* at the age of 18 years by one eminent British colonial servant, Mr T.E. Ravenshaw, may have been a factor in the choice of the college's locality.[412] An education department too was created and placed in charge of Dr H.C. Bowser (or Bowzer) who was at the same time medical officer.[413] Medical expertise appears to have been an appropriate qualification also for educational management. A school was established in the capital, Baripada, and "an English-knowing teacher and an Uriya pandit were placed in charge of it".[414] The main beneficiaries of the amenity would have been members of the better-off Hindu castes, which made up part of the fourteen percent of the state's non-tribal population. The majority of 70 percent aboriginals and semi-aboriginals were described as "very backward" and the logic of *Realpolitik* seems to have suggested that in regard to education and other matters the situation was to remain like this.[415]

Dr Bowser was also in charge of the dispensary, which was described as "charitable", but as it was located within the *Rajbati* or royal palace compound, it was accessible only to the more privileged amongst the state's people, namely those who largely did not have to pay for its maintenance.[416] Like in Travancore and other areas in South Asia, it was reported that "people had no faith" in Western medicine and its practitioners: "very few came to Dr. Bowzer for medical help and ultimately he resigned".[417] And as is documented also for other states, the situation improved when a Hindu, Pravakar Das, referred to as a "hospital assistant", was placed in charge; he "succeeded to some extent in making it popular".[418] The fact that, in addition, "a local native doctor, who dispensed Ayurvedic medicines", was available, may have been crucial.[419]

Given the lack of interest in and demand for 'modern', Western medicine during a period when health reforms were introduced in British-ruled and some other states outside Orissa, the establishment of a lunatic asylum would have been even more out of place. The trappings of modernity in elite Hindu society in Mayurbhanj did not then extend to such private and sensitive matters as one's physical let alone mental health. And in case they did, private consultations and treatment in Calcutta, Cuttack, or Madras could be arranged.[420] In any case, tribals, whose spiritual lives were influenced by "ants, ghosts and whispering trees", were likely to have considered medical and psychiatric treatment and confinement in a Western-style institution as punishment rather than salvation.[421]

In 1882/3, Mr H.P. Wylly wrote in his annual report on the medical department of Mayurbhanj that a new dispensary was to be built as the old one was in a "dilapidated condition".[422] As was the case in other Princely states, taxes were imposed on the general population so that the new facility could be established and newly staffed, as well as the town's "very bad" sanitation improved. People in the *mofussil* or rural areas, who were to pay for these measures, had to make do without and wait until 1910 for what was referred to as "well-equipped dispensaries" in the official reports. Meanwhile, Mr Wylly appointed Dr Purna Chandra Gupta as head of the medical department, but it is not clear if the suggestion of adding a "good assistant surgeon" to the "one hospital assistant, on Rs 40, and a compounder, on Rs 10" was taken up. It is noted though by S.N. Sarkar, in suspiciously overly optimistic terms but without specific evidence, that by 1910 the eight dispensaries in the districts were each headed by "a competent medical officer and provided with an excellent stock of medicines and appliances to provide relief to the thousands who attended them in the course of the year".[423] In a similar vein, the dispensary at Baripada was extended and styled as a hospital to commemorate the reign of King Edward, becoming "a model of what such institutions should be".[424]

Although Baripada had become a "municipality" in 1905, following policies modelled on the Municipality Act in British India that helped improve public health measures, mental health remained excluded from the list of priorities. Again the cost for improvements in the city were largely subsidized "by the State", as the records put it; in other words, the rural working population, in the main Adivasis and Dalits or outcastes, were made to pay for what was styled as a "notably clean and well-ordered town".[425] They also paid the price for the economic modernization of the state that occurred from the beginning of the twentieth century. Gazetteers from this period and the hagiographer of Maharaja Sriram Chandra Bhanja (ruled 1890–1912) proudly reported that "the revenue increased from about four lakhs to over three times that amount".[426] Amongst the profitable investments the usual signifiers of "modern development" and "progress" are listed, including the extraction of iron ore by the Tata Iron and Steel Company at Sakchi, roads, the Baripada Hospital and dispensaries, the police station, 300 jails, 30 inspection bungalows, the high school at Baripada, the Victoria Memorial Institute, railways, and irrigation.[427] That Tata for example made its profit on the basis of forced (*bethi*) and cheap tribal labour and that Adivasis were not compensated for the appropriation of their lands needed for the various infrastructural, industrial, and forestry projects was not considered worth mentioning.[428]

Maharajas' donations for charitable causes, especially if they were in support of those in British-ruled areas, did more to enchant colonial officials than make them question how the moneys were come by. Maharaja Purna Chandra Bhanja (ruled 1920–1928), for example, was reported to have "expressed his greatness" by a range of donations such as Rs 200,000 for Rajkumar College in Raipur; Rs 100,000 for Ravenshaw College, Rs 20,000 for the Medical School, and Rs 13,000 for the Utkal Sahitya Parishad [Orissa Literary Association] Building in British-ruled Cuttack; Rs 10,000 for the Orissa Engineering College in Bihar; and Rs 1,000 for the Countess of Reading's Women's Fund.[429] The maharaja and his biographer appear to have been set on leaving an impression of enlightened benevolence on people outside their own state.

It is clear that although the British censored rulers when riots occurred or the state budget was in arrears, they did not intervene on behalf of exploited tribals and lower castes and outcastes; instead they hailed Mayurbhanj as a "modern" and "progressive" state and honoured it with nine-gun salutes. Yet, the British officials in the state were fully aware of the circumstances, not least because from early on administrative staff such as Ravenshaw and Wylly acted for extended periods as quasi-rulers of the states.[430] Ravenshaw, for example, reported on Srinath Bhanja's (ruled 1863 to 1867) heavy-handed approach to food riots in response to the Naanka Durbikhya or the ninth big famine, of 1866.[431] At the same time Ravenshaw was "unwilling", as a later resident, Nilamani Senapati, put it a century later, "to see starvation" in Mayurbhanj.[432] Ravenshaw had even reported to the Government of Bengal that there were two groups of people in Mayurbhanj, namely "Des log" (or tribals, in this context) and "Hatua" or "Sudros" (various Hindu caste groups who were settled in villages and acquired land that the tribals claimed as theirs).[433] As the former lived from hand to mouth, they were vulnerable to food shortages and scarcity occasioned by hoarding and stockpiling on the part of Hatua. As in British Indian provinces, the underlying dynamics of injustice, exploitation, and oppression were not commented on, nor dealt with; in both regions forced labour and extraction of taxes from the rural population served the "enlightened development" and "economic progress" so cherished by the urban middle classes and elites – British as well as Indian. Tribals were also considered as a convenient and cheap reservoir for labour corps during wars, as in the case of the First World War when Wylly, as advisor of the Court of Ward for Purna Chandra Bhanja Deo (ruled 1920–1928), tried to recruit Santhals and other tribes in May 1917. The ensuing uprising by resisting tribals were quashed with the usual brutality, with the help of "armed police reserves from Orissa and 100 infantry men from Calcutta".[434]

Why is a lengthy account of the economics and politics of exploitation in Mayurbhanj and Dhenkanal called for in a chapter supposedly focused on mental health service provision? In fact it is vitally important. Any social history of mental health and psychiatry worth its salt needs to explain absences and consider the wider socio-political and economic context within which certain aspects did, or failed to, gain prominence. The central issue in the case under analysis is why mental health was not considered relevant even on the levels of ideology, discourse, or mere lip service, while it was hailed in other regions as one of the indicators of a state's modernity. Only if we understand the structural and cultural dynamics that determined which areas of "development" and of "enlightened" governance were seen as vital and which ones were neglected will we be able to identify the reasons for mental health and psychiatry becoming the subjects for attention and intervention – however perfunctory and urban-focused – or, alternatively, for disregard and indifference.

As the situation in Orissa shows, lunatic asylums were not always and necessarily part of the ideological arsenal of progress and manifestations of enlightened and modern development. The educated, settled minority communities in what towns there existed in Princely Orissa were able, if they so wished, to have their ill members sent to institutions in neighbouring British-ruled provinces (such as Cuttack in Orissa; Madras; Calcutta in Bengal, or, later, Ranchi in Bihar), even though evidence suggests that they preferred, on the whole, Ayurvedic regimens.

Tribal people on their part relied on the invocation of deities and spirits, treatment by *ojhas* (diviners, practising 'white' magic), *dans* or *jans* (witches who practised 'black' magic), and herbal prescriptions by *raranics* (medicine men or herbal doctors).[435] The demand for treatment in Western-style institutions for such delicate conditions as mental and spiritual un-ease and suffering was therefore low amongst both tribals and Hindu communities in the rural areas, while the urban elite was comparatively small in numbers. The prominent areas of further development that received attention were therefore those that enabled the profitable extraction of natural resources, namely roads, railways, and irrigation. Mental health and labour laws in contrast were bound to create further expense.

In 1872, Hunter had pointed out that in regard to the public works initiated by 'native' dynasties, "Temples, shrines, and tanks form the sole memorials of their rule."[436] His observation appears to have been correct, highlighting as it does the important role of religion in the legitimation of Princely rule. However, like many historians after him, he contrasted this with what the British achieved in an almost celebratory light, namely that "The British Government has directed its energies to less conspicuous and less ornamental, but more useful enterprises."[437] Foremost amongst these were public embankments, canals, roads, and harbour communication. Who profited from these and who had to pay the price for them has been less often focused on in attempts to highlight what is considered to be the advantages of modernity. As Pati has noted, such projects of enlightened commerce, as well as social welfare measures, were achieved through exploitation, namely forced labour, levies on the poor, and no compensation for the land expropriated.[438]

Conclusion

The Indian states were characterized by great diversity of demographic and cultural conditions, power constellations, and patterns of exclusion of particular communities from access to mental and general health services. In these respects the conditions for the majority of the population were not unlike those prevalent in areas directly ruled by the British. In regard to health services, the juxtaposition of British colonial with Indian governance does not allow us to identify the former exclusively with progress and modernity; nor was medical provision in 'progressive' Indian states consistently 'modern' and 'enlightened'. Different states set different priorities and their position in the league tables of indicators of modernity, such as literacy and hospital beds, changed over the decades, depending on the complex social conditions and strength of political movements that framed mental and general health initiatives at different times. For some rulers and their *darbars* Western modernity and its institutions became prestige projects that served Princely self-aggrandizement and legitimation of their power in the eyes of particular Indian communities. These sat comfortably alongside more conventional initiatives, such as the construction of temples, water reservoirs, and indigenous medicine projects. They had the further advantage of inviting approval on the part of the British and facilitating recognition as 'modern' or 'enlightened', regardless of how elite and town-focused Princely health and welfare measures may have been.

In terms of their impact, mental health initiatives in Travancore were as limited as those in British-ruled areas, with an emphasis on provision being made available only in the capital. The majority of the population relied, as hitherto, for better or worse, on the plural field of healing practices available in different regions, ranging from formal medical systems such as Ayurveda, Unani, and Siddha; pilgrimage to healing temples and shrines; consultation of shamans and exorcists; appeals to deities; use of herbs and minerals; and to care by the family. Medical and psychiatric provision along Western lines was hard to come by in both Princely and British India. Hence social control by means of institutionalization in Western-style facilities was equally limited.

Within the wider historiography of South Asia, writing on the history of Indian states has until recently been seen as a conservative endeavour that focuses on backward regions and on concerns irrelevant to the emergence of modernity in the region. The fact that some authors have tended to glorify certain rulers by means of listing their accomplishments in the 'modern' and 'traditional' sectors of governance in hagiographic accounts has only confirmed this view. The resurgence of writing in a nationalist or regionalist vein that takes on the mantle of anti-colonial history by praising 'firsts' achieved by particular Indian states does not do much to facilitate a critical approach towards both colonial and Princely governance, as it is still in an essentialist way bound up with colonial blueprints of what is to count as enlightened and progressive governance. Most importantly, this kind of approach neglects how 'firsts' were achieved, namely who benefitted from and who paid for them. Historians of health and medicine in particular need to avoid the temptation of writing progressivist, linear histories of great men, great institutions, and great inventions that validate the 'civilizing mission', and of expunging the view and fate of the many and of the marginalized, lest they deservedly fall prey to being judged as watercarriers of conservative history.

Notes

1 Royal Bethlem Hospital Archive, London (henceforth: RBH), Edward Mapother Private Papers, India Report, 1938, 29; 15. Many thanks to Colin Dale, Archivist at the Bethlem Museum, for making the material available to me.
2 RBH, Mapother, 40.
3 *Ibid.*, 35.
4 RBH, Mapother, 35. States like Mewar are still glorified by some as "the oldest ruling dynasty in the world". Like other Rajput Princely states, its people were seen by the British as admirable fighters and as members of a 'martial race'. Irmgard Meininger, *The Kingdom of Mewar: Great Struggles and Glory of the World's Oldest Ruling Dynasty*, New Delhi: D.K. Printworld, 2000.
5 RBH, Mapother, 1938, 35. Much of Mapother's report on his tour of India was based on hearsay or consultation of key informants who invariably tended to belong to the senior ranks of the Indian Medical Service. In regard to Mewar, his report drew largely on the views expressed by Lt Col W.C. Hogg, M.D, IMS, Residency Surgeon, Mewar, Udaipur.
6 Mapother's report on Ceylon was published. His manuscript on Indian institutions is available only in typescript. Even his Ceylon report, which was much better researched, had, as Mills and Jain have noted, very limited impact on government decision making.

J.H. Mills and S. Jain, '"A Disgrace to a Civilised Community": Colonial Psychiatry and the Visit of Edward Mapother to South Asia, 1937–8', in G. Mooney and J. Reinarz (eds.), *Permeable Walls: Historical Perspectives on Hospital and Asylum Visiting*, Amsterdam: Rodopi, 2009.

7 On Mapother, see: E. Jones, 'Aubrey Lewis, Edward Mapother and the Maudsley', *Medical History Supplement*, 22, 2003, 3–38; E. Jones and S. Rahman, 'The Maudsley Hospital and the Rockefeller Foundation: The Impact of Philanthropy on Research and Training', *Journal of the History of Medicine and Allied Sciences*, 64(3), 2009, 273–99; R. Hayward, 'Making Psychiatry English: The Maudsley Hospital and the Munich Model', in Volker Roelcke, Paul J. Weindling, and Louise Westwood (eds.), *International Relations in Psychiatry: Britain, Germany, and the United States Through World War II*, Rochester, NY: University of Rochester Press, 2010, 67–90; E. Jones and S. Rahman, 'Framing Mental Illness, 1923–1939: The Maudsley Hospital and Its Patients', *Social History of Medicine*, 21, 2008, 107–25.

8 Quotes from Mapother, in relation to conditions and staff in British-run institutions. RBH, Mapother, 1, 10.

9 Barbara N. Ramusack, *The New Cambridge History of India: The Indian Princes and Their States*, Cambridge: University Press, 2004, 174.

10 Susan Bayly, 'Hindu Kingship and the Origin of Community: Religion, State and Society in Kerala, 1750–1850', *Modern Asian Studies*, 18, 1984, 186–202.

11 M. Griffith, *India's Princes: Short Life Sketches of the Native Rulers of India*, London: W.H. Allen, 1894, 269.

12 Griffith, *Sketches*, 269.

13 *Ibid.*

14 See for example, Manali Desai, 'Indirect British Rule, State Formation, and Welfarism in Kerala, India, 1860–1957', *Social Science History*, 29(3), 2005, 457–88; 457.

15 Frederick Roberts, *Forty-one Years in India*, London: MacMillan, 1898, 501–2. 1902 [1897], Vol. II, 388.

16 Dewan Nagam Aiya provided Roberts' quote in the 1906 Gazetteer, clearly wishing to allude to the high esteem in which the Maharaja was held. [Dewan] V. Nagam Aiya, *The Travancore State Manual*, Vol. I, Thiruvananthapuram: Kerala Gazetteers, 1999 [first published 1906], 603 (quoting from the 1902 edition of Roberts' book: Roberts, *Forty-One Years*, 388). But, revealingly, the Dewan failed to provide the rest of the sentence he had quoted: "and yet this man was steeped in superstition".

17 Nagam Aiya, *State Manual*, Vol. I, 603.

18 *Ibid.*, 555.

19 Manali Desai, 'Indirect British Rule, State Formation, and Welfarism in Kerala, India, 1860–1957', *Social Science History*, 29(3), 2005, 457–88; 469.

20 Ramusack, *Indian Princes*, 34. On the residency system whereby a British official resided in the princely capital, advising the ruler, see C.A. Bayly, *Indian Society and the Making of the British Empire*, Cambridge: University Press, 1988; Michael Fisher, *Indirect Rule in India: Residents and the Residency System, 1764–1858*, Oxford: University Press, 1991.

21 R.N. Yesudas, *Colonel John Munro in Travancore*, Trivandrum: Kerala Historical Society, 1977.

22 P.K.K. Menon, *The History of the Freedom Movement in Kerala*, Vol. 2, 1885–1938, Trivandrum: Government Press, 1972, 40.

23 Fisher, *Indirect Rule*, 214. See also Yesudas, *Munro*.

24 Kerala State Archives, Thiruvananthapuram (henceforth: KSA), 1843, Cover File 15429, 254. Slavery in Trivandrum. Emancipation of.

25 On Charles Grant see: A.T. Embree, *Charles Grant and the British Rule in India*, London: George Allen & Unwin, 1962.

26 Church Missionary Society, *Missionary Register for 1819*, Vol. 7, London: L.B. Seeley, 1819, 265.

27 P.K.M. Tharakan, 'Socio-economic Factors in Educational Development: Case of Nineteenth-century Travancore', *Economic and Political Weekly*, 19, 1984, 1950–72, 1960.

28 Robin Jeffrey, *The Decline of Nayar Dominance: Society and Politics in Travancore, 1847–1908*, New York: Holmes and Meier.

29 Ramusack, *Indian Princes*, 174.

30 Jeffrey, *Decline*, Chapter 3.

31 *Ibid.*, Chapter 2.

32 Nagam Aiya, *State Manual*, Vol. I, 557. S. Ramanath Aiyer, *A Brief Sketch of Travancore: The Model State of India*, Trevandrum: Western Star Press, 1903.

33 Nagam Aiya, *State Manual*, Vol. I, 556.

34 Aeneas Mcleod Ross. LRCS Edinburgh 1858. Assistant Surgeon. Madras 10.2.1859. Surgeon 10.2. 1871. Appointed Physician to HRH Maharaja of Travancore, 1868. Surgeon Major 1.7.1873. Died at Sikandarabad 1.6.1885.

35 KSA, V.V. Pillay, Dewan Peishkar in charge, Travancore Administrative Report, 1870/1, [no further details], Report on Medical Department by AE. M. Ross, 66.

36 KSA, Pillay, Administrative Report, 1870/1, 66.

37 *Ibid.*, 66.

38 *Ibid.*, 67.

39 *Ibid.*, 67.

40 *Ibid.*, 67.

41 *Ibid.*, 67.

42 KSA, Pillay, Administrative Report, 1870/1, 67. Ross argued: "The tanks [water reservoirs] for instance attached to the principal pagodas, which are now in a most insanitary condition might be periodically drained so as to keep the water, as far as may be, fresh and pure. The neighbourhood of these tanks and of other large sources of water supply might be guarded so as to prevent contamination of the waters, and each house holder might be made responsible for the cleanliness of the street opposite his holding."

43 KSA, Pillay, Administrative Report, 1870/1, 67.

44 S. Mishra, *Pilgrimage, Politics and Pestilence: The Haj From the Indian Subcontinent, 1860–1920*, Delhi: Oxford University Press, 2011; R. Johnson and A. Khalid (eds.), *Public Health in the British Empire: Intermediaries, Subordinates and Public Health Practice, 1850–1960*, New York: Routledge, 2012.

45 KSA, Pillay, Administrative Report, 1870/1, 67.

46 *Ibid.*

47 *Ibid.*

48 Samuel Mateer, *Native Life in Travancore*, New Delhi: Education Services, 1991; London: W.H. Allen & Co., 1883, 357.

49 Mateer, *Native Life*, 357.

50 *Ibid.*

51 KSA, Pillay, Administrative Report, 1870/1, 70.

52 Sources differ on the date of its foundation. The Gazetteer of 1906 refers to the 1840s. However, the official records report the Opening ceremony of the "General Hospital at Trivandrum" to have taken place in 1838. KSA, 1838, Cover File 7261, 189.

53 KSA, Pillay, Administrative Report, 1870/1, 72.

54 *Ibid.*, 70.

55 *Ibid.*, 69.

56 *Ibid.*, 70.

57 A.S. Menon, *Kerala District Gazetteer – Trivandrum*, Trivandrum: Superintendent of Government Press, 1962, 698.

58 KSA, Administration Report, Medical Department, 1935/6. Published 1937, 3. The Nambudiri Brahmins were at the top of the ritual caste hierarchy. Anyone who was not a Nambudiri was considered by them as an untouchable and polluting.

See: E. Kathleen Gough, 'Nayars: Central Kerala', in David Murray Schneider and E. Kathleen Gough, *Matrilineal Kinship*, Berkeley: University of California Press, 1961, 409–414.
59 See debate on Temple Entry Declaration, note 183.
60 KSA, Pillay, Administrative Report, 1870/1, 73.
61 KSA, 1897/8, Cover File, 4520, 126.
62 KSA, Pillay, Administrative Report, 1870/1, 77.
63 *Ibid.*
64 KSA, 1835, Cover File 16237, 135.
65 KSA, 1864–90, Cover File 3013, 556.
66 KSA, 1866, Cover File 15883, 663. 1866, Cover File 15982, 664. 1866, Cover File 16079, 665. 1866, Cover File 16480, 671.
67 KSA, 1867, Cover File 16081, 719. 1871, Cover File 15882, 876. 1869, Cover File 1569, 808. 1867, Cover File 16477, 736. 1869, Cover File 369, 785. 1869, Cover File 16083, 816. 1868, Cover File 52, 738.
68 KSA, Pillay, Administrative Report, 1870/1, 77–82.
69 *Ibid.*, 77–82.
70 *Ibid.*, 82–3.
71 KSA, 1875–95, Cover File 15049, 1095.
72 KSA, 1879, Cover File 16174, 2039. 1881–85, Cover File 3118, 2111.
73 KSA, 1884, Cover File 15860, 2351.
74 For example, KSA, 1890, Cover File 910, 2959. 1892, Cover File 682, 3215.
75 KSA, 1892, Cover File 10168, 333.
76 KSA, 1896, Cover File 8340, 3970. See also, on the organization and re-organization of the Medical Department: 1898, Cover File 15157, 4537. 1898, Cover File 15876, 4558.
77 Mateer, *Native Life*, 351.
78 *Ibid.*, 370.
79 *Ibid.*, 370.
80 KSA, Administration Report, 1870/1, 66.
81 *Ibid.*, 90.
   The figures displayed in this table do not include all expenses, as the maintenance of buildings, for example, was listed under the contingency fund. So was an extra supply of "medicines, diet etc for the Hospitals" on account of the extended operations of the Medical Department referred to earlier by court physician Ross, and "a supply of Medical Stores having been procured from Europe, calculated to last more than one year". These charges amounted to about Rs 30,000.
   KSA, Administration Report, 1870/1, 128.
82 KSA, Administration Report, 1870/1, 99.
83 KSA, Administration Report, 1870/1, 123. *see note 81, above.
84 On the importance of religious institutions in the legitimation of Princely rule, see Chapters 3 and 4 by Biswamoy Pati.
85 National Library, Kolkata, *A Handbook of Travancore, Containing Every Information About the Country, Its People, Geography, Government, History etc.* (Trevandrum [n.p.] 1881), Vol. 1, 286.
86 Dick Kooiman, *Conversion and Social Equality in India: The London Missionary Society in Southern Travancore*, Delhi: Manohar, 1989; Jeffrey Cox, *Imperial Fault Lines: Christianity and Colonial Power in India, 1818–1940*, Stanford: University Press, 2002.
87 R.N. Yesudas, *The History of the London Missionary Society in Travancore, 1806–1908*, Trivandrum: Kerala History Society, 1980, 5.
88 I.H. Hacker, *A Hundred Years in Travancore, 1806–1906*, London: H.R. Allenson, 1908, 24. Jeffrey quoted a LMS missionary who noted that although conversion of all strata amongst Hindus were aspired to, it was mainly untouchables who were attracted

by the hope that "their material grievances are more speedily, effectually and cheaply redressed by making the missionary their friend than in any other way." Jeffrey, *Decline*, 39. Also, conversion rates increased during famine years, as in 1810–1812, and changes in the liability for poll tax, too, affected conversion. Kooiman refers to the fluctuating conversion rates and changes in religious denomination in hours of need as a "rush hour in an already existing religious boundary traffic". Koiman, *Conversion*, 82; see also pp. 72–3.

89 Mateer, *Native Life*, 353. Chapter titled "Recent Measures of Reform".
90 KSA, 1853, Cover File 16075, 411.
91 KSA, 1845, Cover File 15335, 312.1872, Cover File 15311, 932. 1874, Cover File 15304, 1034.
92 Mateer, *Native Life*, 357.
93 *Ibid.*, 359.
94 T.C. Varghese, *Agrarian Change and Economic Consequences: Land Tenures in Kerala, 1850–1960*, Bombay: Allied Pres, 1970.
95 K.P. Kannan, *Of Rural Proletarian Struggles: Mobilization and Organization of Rural Workers in South-West India*, Delhi: Oxford University Press, 1988, 40–50.
96 Jeffrey, *Decline*.
97 Koji Kawashima, *Missionaries and a Hindu State: Travancore, 1858–1936*, Delhi: Oxford University Press, 1998, Chapter 6; Jeffrey, *Decline*, Chapters 3 to 5.
98 See on this aspect, for example, P. Chandramohan, 'Popular Culture and Socio-religious Reform: Narayana Guru and the Ezhavas of Travancore', *Studies in History*, 3, 1987, 57–74; P.K.K. Menon, *The History of the Freedom Movement in Kerala*. Vol. 2, 1885–1938, Trivandrum: Government Press, 1972.
99 See, in regard to the former, T.K. Ravindran, *Asan and Social Revolution in Kerala: A Study of His Assembly Speeches*, Trivandrum: Kerala Historical Society, 1972. See also Menon, *Freedom Movement*.
100 As Kent has pointed out, Mateer translated the term *dharmabhumi* as "land of charity", curtailing the meaning of *dharma* to the Christian connotation of charity. E.F. Kent, 'Books and Bodices. Material Culture and Protestant Missions in Colonial South Asia', 67–88, in J.S. Scott and G. Griffith (eds.), *Mixed Messages. Materiality, Textuality, Missions*, London: Palgrave Macmillan, 2005, 76.
101 Kooiman, *Conversion*.
102 Kawashima, *Missionaries*.
103 The Education Code of 1909 enabled government to exert control over education.
104 Desai, 'Indirect British Rule', 473.
105 J.H. Hutton, *Census of India 1931* Part 1. Report 1, New Delhi: Office of the Registrar General, 1933, 326.
106 Desai, 'Indirect British Rule', 474.
107 Susan Bayly, *Saints, Goddesses and Kings: Muslims and Christians in South Indian Society, 1700–1900*, Cambridge: University Press, 1976.
108 Nicholas B. Dirks, *The Hollow Crown: Ethnohistory of an Indian Kingdom*, New York: Cambridge University Press, 1987, and Castes *of Mind*, Princeton University Press, 2001.
109 Kawashima, *Missionaries*, 18–23.
110 Ramusack, *Princes*, 178.
111 [Dewan] V. Nagam Aiya, *The Travancore State Manual*, Vol. III, Thiruvananthapuram: Kerala Gazetteers, 1999 [first published 1906], 521.
112 Nagam Aiya, *State Manual*, Vol. III, 521.
113 Nagam Aiya, *State Manual*, Vol. III, 521. On *Sirkar Devaswam Pattom*, see 331–2, 324–5.
114 Nagam Aiya, *State Manual*, Vol. III, 521.
115 *Ibid.*, 521.
116 *Ibid.*, 521.

117 *Ibid.*, 524.
118 *Ibid.*, 521–2.
119 *Ibid.*, 524.
120 *Ibid.*, 524.
121 *Ibid.*, 524.
122 *Ibid.*, 241.
123 *Ibid.*, 525.
124 *Ibid.*, 525.
125 *Ibid.*, 526.
126 *Ibid.*, 526.
127 Nagam Aiya, *State Manual*, Vol. I, 537.
128 S. Mateer, *"The Land of Charity:" A Descriptive Account of Travancore and Its People, With Especial Reference to Missionary Labour*, London: Snow and Co., 1871 [1870].
129 Nagam Aiya, *State Manual*, Vol. III, 525.
130 Nagam Aiya, *State Manual*, Vol. III, 525. Quotation from the deeds of the Raja of Paroor (Parur).
131 Nagam Aiya, *State Manual*, Vol. III, 525.
132 Napier quote in Nagam Aiya, *State Manual*, Vol. I, 555.
133 *Ibid.*
134 Nagam Aiya, *State Manual*, Vol. I, 619.
135 K.N. Panikkar, *Culture, Ideology, Hegemony. Intellectuals and Social Consciousness in Colonial India*, London: Anthem, 2002 [1995], 152.
136 Panikkar, *Culture*, 152. On the revival of indigenous medical tradition amongst the Ezhava under colonialism and its interconnection with caste mobilization, see: Burton Cleetus, 'Subaltern Medicine and Social Mobility: The experience of the Ezhava in Kerala', *Indian Anthropologist*, 37(1), 2007, 147–72.
137 [Dewan] V. Nagam Aiya, *The Travancore State Manual*, Vol. II, Thiruvananthapuram: Kerala Gazetteers, 1999 [first published 1906], 545.
138 Nagam Aiya, *State Manual*, Vol. II, 545. Each received the tidy sum of Rs 35 per month as a honorarium.
139 Nagam Aiya, *State Manual*, Vol. II, 545.
140 *Ibid.*, 546.
141 *Ibid.*, 546.
142 Nagam Aiya, *State Manual*, Vol. II, 546. *Ashtanga Hridayam* refers to an approach and a Sanskrit text, the *Ashtanga Hridayam Samhita,* from 500 C.E., compiled by Vagbhata.
143 *Ibid.*, 546.
144 *Ibid.*, 546.
145 *Ibid.*, 546.
146 *Ibid.*, 546.
147 Nagam Aiya, *State Manual*, Vol. II, 546. Reference to Administration Report for 1066 M.E., Report on the Travancore Census of 1891.
148 Nagam Aiya, *State Manual*, Vol. II, 546.
149 *Ibid.*, 546.
150 *Ibid.*, 547.
151 Nagam Aiya, *State Manual*, Vol. II, 547. Reference to Administration Report for 1066 M.E., Report on the Travancore Census of 1891.
152 Nagam Aiya, *State Manual*, Vol. II, 547. It was not specified if this sum related to Western medicine or to Vaidyasalas; it is likely that it was the former. Although comparisons over time, place, and nomenclature are problematic, it is intriguing to note that in the twenty-first century, the Indian Union spends about 4.1 percent of GDP on healthcare, the UK 9.6 percent, and Germany 11.6 percent.
153 Nagam Aiya, *State Manual*, Vol. II, 547.

154 Menon, *Gazetteer – Trivandrum*, 672.
155 *Ibid.*, 672.
156 *Ibid.*, 673.
157 KSA, 1928, File 31, 1595/28.
158 Menon, *Gazetteer – Trivandrum*, 711.
159 *Ibid.*
160 Panikkar, *Culture*, 162–7. Vaidya Chintamani Joshi, 'A Life of Healing: A Biography of Vaidya P.S. Varrier', *Journal of Ayurveda and Integrative Medicine*, 2, 2011, 35–6.
161 Panikkar, *Culture*, 162, 167–8.
162 *Ibid.*, 168.
163 KSA, Administration Report of the Medical Department, 1942/3, Trivandrum: Government Press, 1944, II.
164 KSA, Administration Report of the Medical Council 1946/7, Trivandrum: Government Press, 1948, 1.
165 KSA, Administration Report, 1946/7, 1.
166 *Ibid.*, 2.
167 *Ibid.*, 2.
168 *Ibid.*, 2.
169 *Ibid.*, I.
170 *Ibid.*, 2.
171 KSA, Report on the Administration of Travancore for the year 1904/5, Trivandrum: Travancore Government Press, 1905, 57. In 1905, there were 23 hospitals and 21 dispensaries in the state.
172 KSA, Report on Administration, 1904/5, 58.
173 *Ibid.*
174 KSA, Report on Administration, Vital Statistics, Vaccination and Medical Services, 1906/7, Trivandrum: Government Press, 1907, Appendix XXI, lviii–lix.
175 KSA, Report on Administration, 1906/7, Appendix XXI, lviii–lix.
176 In order to gauge the magnitude of the funds made available for healthcare, they again need to be set against expenses incurred in other areas, such as, for example:

Devaswom or Religious Institutions	Rs 901,779
Oottupurahs or Charitable Institutions	Rs 510,522
Subsidy to British Government	Rs 810,878
Maharajah's Tour to Madras	Rs 55,618

KSA, Report on Administration, 1906/7, Appendix XXI, lviii–lix.
177 KSA, Administration Report, Medical Department, 1935/6. Published 1937, 14; KSA, Administration Report 1946/7, 14.
178 KSA, Administration Report, Medical Department, 1934/5. Published 1936, 16.
179 Percentages have been calculated by the author.
KSA, Administration Report, Medical Department, 1935/6. Published 1937, 15. KSA, Administration Report, 1946/7, 15. No report for the year 1121 was available at KSA; the figures for this year are taken from the report of 1122, which referred back to 1121.
180 In 1944/5, 40 percent of patients were listed as "other classes". The following year, 21 percent were in this category, while 20 percent were designated as "Christians". Census numbers amounted to 32 percent for Christians.
181 Hutton, Census of India, 1931, Appendix I, 471.
182 *Ibid.*
183 R. Jeffrey, 'Temple-Entry Movement in Travancore, 1860–1940', *Social Scientist*, 4(8), 1976, 3–27; C.K. Pullapilly, 'The Ishavas of Kerala and Their Historic Struggle for Acceptance in the Hindu society', *Journal of Asian and African Studies*, 11(1), 1976, 24–36; L. Ouwerkerk, *No Elephants for the Maharaja: Social and Political Change in the Princely State of Travancore, 1921–1947*, New Delhi: Manohar, 1994.

184 Hutton, India Census 1931, Appendix 1, Table B.
185 Census Data for 1900/1 indicate the same figure for Muslims, namely seven percent. Hindu: 69 percent, Christian: 24 percent, Animism: 1 percent, Others: 0.01 percent. Overall population: *ca.* 3 Mio.
186 1931: 2,497,000 men; 2,463,000 women; 1941: 3,045,000 men; 3,025,000 women.
187 Percentages have been calculated by the author.
    KSA, Administration Report, Medical Department, 1935/6. Published 1937, 14; KSA, Administration Report of the Medical Council 1946/7, Trivandrum: Government Press, 1948, 14. Children were listed separately, but not segregated by gender: 1935: 639.091; 1945: 577, 818.
188 For more detail, see R. Jeffrey, 'Women and the "Kerala Model". Four Lives, 1870s-1980s', *Journal of South Asian Studies*, 12(2), 1989, 13–32.
189 K. Rajasekharan Nair, 'A Pioneer in Medicine – Dr Mary Poonan Lukose', *Samyukta: A Journal of Women's Studies*, 2(2), 2002, 117–21. For an account based on this source, see K.S. Mohindra, [no title], *Hektoen International: A Journal of Medical Humanities*, 7(4), 2015 – online source.
190 C. Hayavadana Rao, *The Indian Biographical Dictionary*, Madras: Pillar, 1915, 330.
191 Lakshmi Raghunandan, *At the Turn of the Tide: The Life and Times of Maharani Setu Lakshmi Bayi: The Last Queen of Travancore*, Bangalore: Maharani Setu Lakshmi Bayi Memorial Charitable Trust, 1995, 133.
192 Raghunandan, *Turn of the Tide*, 133.
193 *Ibid.*
194 KSA: Administration Report, Medical Department, 1933/4, published 1935, 1. In 1932/3 Lukose was appointed as acting durbar physician, then as deputy durbar physician (alongside Dr W.A. Noble), to assist Dr B.L. Salter/Slater, MBBS, MRCS, LRCP (London), the *darbar* physician. KSA, Administration Report, Medical Department, 1932/3. Published 1934, i.
195 KSA: Administration Report, Medical Department 1937/8, published in 1939, I.
196 W. Ernst, 'The Indianization of Colonial Medicine', *NTM – Journal for the History of Science, Technology and Medicine*, 20(4), 2012, 61–89.
197 On medical training and fight for positions by women see: Ellen S. More, *Restoring the Balance: Women Physicians and the Profession of Medicine, 1850–1995*, Cambridge, MA: Harvard University Press, 1999.
198 KSA, Administration Report, 1946/7, 32.
199 W. Ernst, *Colonialism and Transnational Psychiatry: The Development of an Indian Mental Hospital in British India, c. 1925–1940*, London: Anthem, 2013.
200 KSA, *Administration Report*, 1946/7, 32.
201 *Ibid.*, 32.
202 *Ibid.*, 32.
203 KSA, Pillay, Administrative Report, 1870/1, 74.
204 *Ibid.*, 74.
205 Menon, *Gazetteer – Trivandrum*, 708.
206 KSA, Pillay, *Administrative Report*, 1870/1, 74–5.
207 *Ibid.*, 74.
208 *Ibid.*, 74.
209 *Ibid.*, 75.
210 *Ibid.*, 75.
211 *Ibid.*, 75.
212 *Ibid.*, 76.
213 On the role of work in psychiatry, see: W. Ernst (ed.), *Work, Psychiatry and Society, c. 1750–2000*, Manchester: University Press, 2016.
214 KSA, Pillay, Administrative Report, 1870/1, 75–6.

215 On patient work in British India, see W. Ernst, "'Useful Both to the Patients as Well as to the State." Patient Work in Colonial Mental Hospitals in South Asia, c. 1818–1948', in Ernst (ed.) *Work*.
216 See for example P. Michael, *Care and Treatment of the Mentally Ill in North Wales, 1800–2000*, Cardiff: University of Wales Press, 2003.
217 KSA: Pillay, Administrative Report, 1870/1, 74.
218 KSA, Pillay, Administrative Report, 1870/1, 75. The position of Dewan Peishkar was equivalent to that of District Collector in British India.
219 KSA, Pillay, Administrative Report, 1870/1, 75.
220 P. Chandramohan, 'Popular Culture and Socio-religious Reform: Narayana Guru and the Ezhavas of Travancore', *Studies in History*, 3, 1987, 57–74.
221 KSA, Pillay, Administrative Report, 1870/1, 75.
222 *Ibid.*
223 *Ibid.*
224 KSA, 1877, Cover File 1162, 607.
225 T.K. Velu Pillai, *The Travancore State Manual*, Vol. IV, Trivandrum: Government of Travancore, 1940, 217.
226 KSA, 1880–1883, Cover File 4162, 82.
227 *Ibid.*
228 *Ibid.*
229 For example, see W. Ernst, *Colonialism and Transnational Psychiatry*.
230 KSA, 1880–1883, Cover File 4162, 82.
231 *Ibid.*
232 *Ibid.*
233 *Ibid.*
234 Esmonde White was in charge of drawing up the new Civil Medical Code, which was approved by the government in 1897/8. KSA, 1897/8., Cover File 4520, 122.
235 KSA, 1889, Cover File 3634, 2886. Durbar Physician Office to Dewan, 20.9.1889.
236 KSA, 1889, Cover File 3634, 2886. Petition to Dewan, 31 Avani 1065.
237 KSA, 1889, Petition to Dewan.
238 *Ibid.*
239 *Ibid.*
240 KSA, 1889, Cover File 3634, 2886. Durbar Physician to Dewan, 7.10.1889.
241 KSA, 1889, Durbar Physician to Dewan.
242 *Ibid.*
243 *Ibid.*
244 See on debates on 'wrongful confinement' during the nineteenth century: Peter McCandless, 'Liberty and Lunacy: The Victorians and Wrongful Confinement', *Journal of Social History*, 11(3), 1978, 366–86.
245 KSA, 1889, Durbar Physician to Dewan.
246 KSA 1889, Cover File 3634, 2886, Dewan to Durbar Physician, 5.10.1889.
247 KSA 1889, Cover File 3634, 2886. Note to Dewan, appended to Durbar Physician to Dewan, 7.10.1889.
248 KSA, 1889, Cover File 3634, 2886. Secretary to Dewan to Petitioner, 27.10.1889.
249 KSA, 1888, Cover File 2764, 2715.
250 KSA, 1880–1883, Cover File 4162, 82.
251 KSA, 1896, Cover File 3636, 152. Letter by C.F. Breay, 17.1.1895.
252 KSA, 1896, Cover File 3636, 152. Chief Engineer to Dewan, 26.5.1896.
253 KSA, 1896, Cover File 3636, 152. Chief Engineer to Dewan, 26.5.1896. If the bungalow was made available for "the use of any European official", Jopp pointed out, it "would at once become impossible for any officers of superior service to make use of it".
254 KSA, Report 1904/5, Appendix, iv.

255 KSA, 1896, Cover File 3636, 152. Mr La Bouchiere to Dewan, 29.4.1896.
256 KSA, 1896, Cover File 3636, 152. Dewan to Chief Engineer, 8.5.1896.
257 Nagam Aiya, *State Manual*, Vol. II, 499.
258 *Ibid.*, 499.
259 *Ibid.*, 524.
260 *Ibid.*, 524.
261 *Ibid.*, 524.
262 KSA, Report on Administration, Vital Statistics, Vaccination and Medical Services, 1899/1900, Trivandrum: Government Press, 1901, 91.
263 KSA, Report on Administration, 1899/1900, 91, 93.
264 *Ibid.*, 92.
265 Nagam Aiya, *State Manual*, Vol. II, 522.
266 *Ibid.*, 522.
267 *Ibid.*, 522, Table VIII.
268 *Ibid.*, 523.
269 *Ibid.*, 523.
270 Anne Digby, 'Woman's Biological Straitjacket', in Susan Mendas and Jane Randall (eds.), *Sexuality and Subordination: Interdisciplinary Studies of Gender in the Nineteenth Century*, New York: Routledge, 1989, 192–220.
271 Nagam Aiya, *State Manual*, Vol. II, 523.
272 *Ibid.*, 523.
273 *Ibid.*, 500.
274 *Ibid.*, 524.
275 KSA, Report on Administration, 1899/1900, 94.
276 *Ibid.*, 94.
277 *Ibid.*, 95.
278 *Ibid.*, 95.
279 Nagam Aiya, *State Manual*, Vol. II, 536. There also existed four bi-weekly dispensaries and six weekly dispensaries in Travancore.
280 KSA, Report on Administration, 1899/1900, 126.
281 KSA, Report on Administration, 1899/1900, 94. For example, Thomson kept a "close check" on the procurement of drugs and instruments, cancelling the purchase of rarely used patent medicines and drugs.
282 KSA, Report 1904/5, 56.
283 *Ibid.*
284 KSA, Report on Administration, 1899/1900, 98.
285 KSA, [G.T. MacKenzie, Resident in Travancore and Cochin], *Administrative Report and Budget Estimates [1899/1900 and 1901/1902 respectively]*, Madras: Superintendent, Government Press, 1901, 8.
286 KSA, MacKenzie, *Budget Estimates*, 8.
287 KSA, Report 1904/5, 51.
288 KSA, Review of the Administration Report, Resident to Chief Secretary of Government, 29 January 1906, 3.
289 KSA, Review, 29 January 1906, 3.
290 KSA, Review, 29 January 1906, 4 The reforms included the reorganization of the Settlement Department; creation of a separate Revenue Department under an Excise Commissioner; reform of the finance system; and the reorganization of the Huzur (legislative) office system. P. 6.
291 KSA, Review, 29 January 1906, 5.
292 KSA, Report 1904/5, Appendix, xxxiv. According to Velu Pillai, patients were transferred from the old buildings to Oolampara between 1903 and 1904. T.K. Velu Pillai, *The Travancore State Manual*, Vol. IV, Trivandrum: Government of Travancore, 1940, 217.
293 Velu Pillai, *State Manual*, Vol. IV, 218.

294 *Ibid.*
295 *Ibid.*
296 *Ibid.*
297 KSA, Administration Report, Medical Department, 1928/9. Published 1929. P. 4.
298 KSA, Administration Report, Medical Department, 1930/1. Published 1932. P. 7.
299 KSA, Administration Report, Medical Department, 1931/2. Published 1933.
300 KSA, Administration Report, 1931/2.
301 *Ibid.*, 7.
302 KSA, Administration Report, 1932/3, 5. KSA, Administration Report 1933/4, 17.
303 KSA, Administration Report 1933/4, 17.
304 KSA, Administration Report 1933/4, 17. Unlike other institutional reports that year, the sections on the mental hospital were published with an unusually large number of typing errors. These have been corrected by the author to avoid a frequent use of square brackets in original citations.
305 KSA, Administration Report 1933/4, 17.
306 KSA, 1901, File 10166, 5191. 1902, File 10205, 5501. Later, a weaver was mentioned, who was then apparently attached to the Hospitals at Oolampara, i.e. the leper and mental hospitals and the hospital for chronic diseases. KSA, Administration Report, 1933/4, 4.
307 KSA, Administrative Report, 1900, 98.
308 KSA, Administration Report, 1928/9, 11.
309 KSA, Administration Report, 1933/4, 17.
310 *Ibid.*
311 *Ibid.*
312 *Ibid.*
313 Voluntary boarders were to be encouraged, following "amendments in Lunacy Regulation of 1080 [1904/5] . . . pending consideration of Government".
     KSA, Administration Report, 1934/5, 23. The Lunacy Regulation of 1904/5 laid down the procedures and responsibilities for the admission and confinement of "dangerous lunatics" only. The Lunacy Regulation of 1935 was to be based on the Indian Lunacy Act of 1912, which was in force in British Indian provinces and allowed for, amongst other things, the admission of voluntary boarders.
314 KSA, Administration Report, 1933/4, 17.
315 KSA, Administration Report, 1934/5, 23.
316 Johnson gained full charge of the Mental Hospital on the transfer to the District Hospital at Changanacherry of the previous postholder when the Leper Hospital and the Hospital for Chronic Diseases were removed from Oolumpara. KSA, Administration Report, 1934/5, i.
317 KSA, Administration Report, 1934/5, 23.
318 KSA, Administration Report, 1935/6, 4.
319 KSA, Administration Report, 1935/6, p 11. There were a total of 127 nurses in the state. However, none was assigned to the mental hospital.
320 KSA, Administration Report, 1934/5, I.
321 *Ibid.*, 10.
322 *Ibid.*, 10.
323 *Ibid.*, 10.
324 *Ibid.*, 10.
325 *Ibid.*, 10.
326 KSA, Administration Report, 1934/5, 10. The practice of warning the public of potential fraud has been retained. For example, in the entrance hall of the Kerala State Archives, a notice says that staff are not allowed to accept gratuities. The notice might explain why the author was unable to assess a series of documents that apparently were no longer available although they had been listed in the catalogue. The same problem prevailed at the Mysore Archives – albeit no warning notice was displayed there.

327 KSA, Administration Report, Medical Department, 1939/40. Published 1941, 1.
328 KSA, Administration Report, 1942/3, 6. Towards the war, a means-tested levy was introduced for medicines and medical attendance except surgical operations to those whose monthly income was Rs 50 and above. KSA, Administration Report, 1946/7, 5.
329 KSA, Administration Report 1942/3, II.
330 *Ibid.*, 9.
331 KSA, Administration Report, Medical Department, 1936/7. Published 1938, 15.
332 KSA, Administration Report, 1937/8, 7.
333 KSA, Administration Report, Medical Department, 1943/4. Published 1945, I.
334 KSA, Administration Report, 1946/7, 11. The categories for nurses consisted of European nursing sister; Indian nursing sisters; staff nurses; higher trained nurses; other nurses (male, female); sick nurses. It is not clear whether those at the mental hospital were specially trained mental health nurses or relatively poorly trained ones.
335 KSA, Administration Report 1942/3, I.
336 Mr V. Kumara Pillai MBBS, FRCP&S was promoted from first grade assistant surgeon to second grade deputy surgeon on 19 Kumbhom 1119 [1944]. KSA, Administration Report, 1943/4, 8.
337 KSA, Administration Report 1946/7, 31–2.
338 E.R. Brown, 'Public Health in Imperialism: Early Rockefeller Programs at Home and Abroad', *American Journal of Public Health*, 66(9), 1976, 897–903; E.R. Brown, *Rockefeller Medicine Men: Medicine and Capitalism in America*, Berkeley: University of California Press, 1979.
339 KSA, Administration Report 1946/7, 7. On the eve of Indian Independence, Pillai handed over his duties at the Mental Hospital to Assistant Surgeon A. Kasim Pillay. KSA, Administration Report 1946/7, 31–2.
340 See, for example, the case of Dr J.E. Dhunjibhoy, in W. Ernst, '"Colonial" and "Modern" Psychiatry in British India: Treatments at the Indian Mental Hospital at Ranchi, 1925–1940', in W. Ernst and T. Mueller (eds.), *Transnational Psychiatries*, Newcastle: Cambridge Scholars, 2010, 80–115.
341 I owe this information on the transnational history of the Meyer classification scheme to Professor German Berrios, to whom many thanks for his generous help are due. On Meyer's impact on psychiatrists' clinical skills, see: S. Lamb, 'Social Skills: Adolf Meyer's Revision of Clinical Skill for the New Psychiatry of the Twentieth Century', *Medical History*, 59(3), 2015, 443–64.
342 According to Berrios, psychiatrist and anthropologist Morris Carstairs was also important in this regard. He had been born and brought up in Mussoorie, in British India, spoke Hindi fluently, and after being a disciple of Aubrey Lewis at Maudsley Hospital London became Professor at Edinburgh in 1961. Many an Indian psychiatrist came to train in his department where Meyer's classification happened to be the official one – introduced by D.K. Henderson himself who held the Edinburgh chair between 1932 and 1954.
343 KSA, Administration Report, Medical Department, 1944/5. Published 1946, pp. 26–29.
344 KSA, Administration Report, Medical Department, 1944/5, Trivandrum: Government Press, 1946, 24.
345 KSA, Administration Report 1944/5, 24.
346 KSA, Administration Report 1946/7, 33.
347 At the time of writing, the Osler Library at McGill University displayed images on Light Therapeutics, c. 1901–1944. Not much appears to have been written about the history of the application of light treatment in psychiatry. For twentieth-century developments, see: S. Carter, 'The Medicalization of Sunlight in the Early Twentieth Century', *Journal of Historical Sociology*, 25, 2012, 83–105.
348 KSA, Administration Report 1946/7, 33. The table was titled, "X-Ray Exposure", but this was clearly an error. The report on the Tuberculosis Hospital, Nagercoil, which followed the Mental Hospital Report, shows that the usual format was to report on how many patients were treated in the X-Ray Department, which was responsible for X-ray examinations as well as light treatment.

349 KSA, Administration Report 1946/7, 33.
350 See the range of recreation pursuits offered to inmates at the Ranchi Indian Mental Hospital in British-ruled India. W. Ernst, *Colonialism and Transnational Psychiatry: The Development of an Indian Mental Hospital in British India, c. 1925–1940*, London: Anthem, 2013.
351 KSA, Administration Report 1946/7, 33.
352 Travancore's Dewan Sir C.P. Ramaswami Iyer promoted the idea that after Britain's withdrawal from the Subcontinent, Travancore should become an independent country, following the American model. After lengthy negotiations, Travancore eventually joined the Indian Union in 1949.
353 Numbers based on annual administrative reports, selected on the basis of availability of comparative data.
354 Dr Gopalakrishnan Peedikayil, MBBS (Kerala), DPM (NIMHANS), MRCPsych (London), formerly Additional Director of Health Services Department, Kerala and Superintendent and Head of the Department of Psychiatry in Mental Health Centres in Kerala. *Some Paths Treaded On* http://pngsblogs.blogspot.co.uk/2014/12/some-paths-treaded-on.html (accessed on 28 January 2016). Peedikayil issued what he calls "The Hospital Entry Proclamation 1985", allowing people to see and live with their unwell relatives. He reports that in 1985, 437 out of 998 inmates were found perfectly sane and released from the 510 bedded hospitals without beds (140 patients had been found in a 20 "bedded" ward without beds).
355 Isabelle von Bueltzingsloewen, 'Starvation in French Asylums During the German Occupation (1940–1945): Methodological Issues in a Comparative Historical Investigation', in Ernst and Mueller (eds.), *Transnational Psychiatries*. Max Lafont referred to the event as "mild extermination": Max Lafont, *L'extermination douce. La mort de 40.000 malades mentaux dans les hôpitaux psychiatriques en France, sous le régime de Vichy*, Nantes: Editions de l'AREFPPI, 1987.
356 The particular years for presentation in Figures 5.4, 5.5, 5.6, and 5.7 in this section have been selected on the basis of the completeness of data available in the Cover Files and Administrative Reports over the period identified. Mortality data are available for more years than are shown in Figure 5.3, and, as Figure 5.6 indicates, considerable fluctuation was present. However, the trendline still indicates an increase in deaths over time, mainly due to the higher figures towards the end of the period.

Figure 5.6 Percentage of patients who died, of total number treated during the year, with trendline, 1897–1947

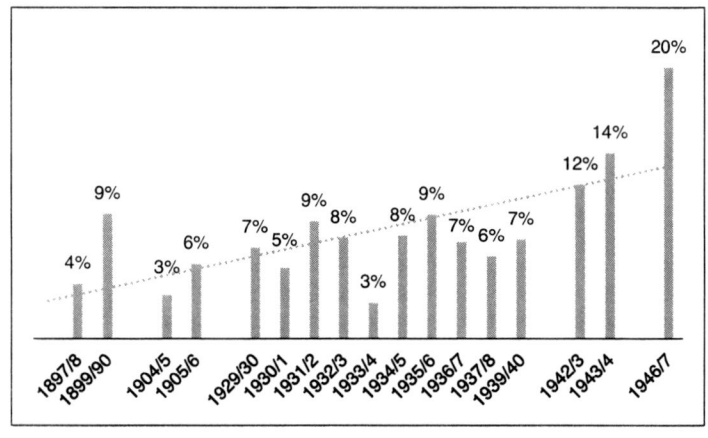

Calculated from Cover Files and Administrative Reports.

357 See Ernst, *Colonialism and Transnational Psychiatry.*
358 KSA, Administration Report 1946/7, 15.
359

Figure 5.7 Number of patients admitted, 1897–1947

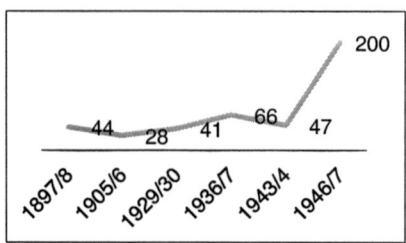

Calculated from Cover Files and Administrative Reports.

360 Data calculated from Cover Files and Administrative Reports.
361 Calculated from Cover Files and Administrative Reports.
362 This report was mentioned but not provided in the regular administration reports of the medical department.
363 RBH, Mapother, 40.
364 *Ibid.*
365 RBH, Mapother, 10.
366 S.P. Sharma, *Three Years in Orissa*, Calcutta: Thacker Spink &Co, 1942, II.
367 Sharma, *Three Years*, II–Iv.
368 *Ibid.*, IV.
369 *Ibid.*, V.
370 P.K. Mishra (ed.), *Comprehensive History and Culture of Orissa*, New Delhi: Kaveri Books, 1997; B. Pati, *Situating Social History: Orissa (1880–1997)*, Hyderabad: Orient Longman, 2001.
371 D.P. Mishra, *People's Revolt in Orissa: A Study of Talcher*, New Delhi: Atlantic, 1998; Biswamoy Pati, 'Interrogating Stereotypes: Exploring the Princely States in Colonial Orissa', *South Asia Research*, 25(2), 2005, 165–82.
372 Pati notes that *bethi* was formally abolished in 1923 and a cess imposed in lieu in the wake of increased monetization during the twentieth century. However, the practice seems to have continued and was noted also by Sharma in the 1940s. Pati, 'Interrogating Stereotypes', 172–3. Sharma, *Three Years*, 42.
373 Pati, 'Interrogating Stereotypes', 173.
374 The term feudal as used here does not mean any implied similarity with Mughal feudalism or medieval European feudalism. See A.L. Basham, *The Wonder That Was India*, London: Sidgwick & Jackson, 1967, 95. "India never had a true feudal system . . . Ancient India had, however, a system of overlordship which was quasi-feudal . . . the Indian system differed from that of Europe in that the relations of overlord and vassal were not regularly based on contract."
375 Sharma, *Three Years*, V. On prajamandal and other movements, see: Sadasiba Pradhan, *Agrarian and Political Movements: States of Orissa, 1931–1949*, New Delhi: Inter-India Publications, 1986; Biswamoy Pati, *Peasants, Tribals and the National Movement in Orissa, 1920–50*, Manohar: New Delhi, 1993.
376 *Praja*: subject, community, public: *mandal*: local administrative division; not quite the same as "county" or "district".
377 W.W. Hunter, *A Statistical Account of Bengal*, Vol. XIX District of Puri and the Orissa Tributary States, London: Truebner, 1877, 6. Hunter went to point out that "The natural difficulties of communication have, so far, shut off the mineral resources of the region from the approach of European capital."

378 L.K. Mahapatra, 'Ex-Princely States of Orissa: Their Social History', in P.K. Mishra (ed.), *Comprehensive History and Culture of Orissa*, Vol. 2, New Delhi: Kaveri, 1997, 896–927.
379 W.W. Hunter, *Orissa, or the Vicissitudes of an Indian Province Under Native and British Rule*, Vol. 2. Appendix IV, London: Elder, 1872, 103. During this period there were only 19 principalities, with a population of about 1 million.
380 Hunter, *Orissa*, 157.
381 *Ibid.*
382 Hunter, *Orissa*, 157. For similar observations in British provinces see Ira Klein, 'Death in India, 1871–1921', *Journal of Asian Studies*, 23(4), 1973, 639–59. Arnold's later study has drawn on Klein's evidence, in particular in relation to smallpox and the goddess *sitala*.
383 Biswamoy Pati, 'The Order of Legitimacy: Princely Orissa, 1850–1947', in Waltraud Ernst and Biswamoy Pati (eds.), *India's Princely States: People, Princes and Colonialism*, London: Routledge, 2007, 85–98.
384 The Bhramaramari plant is connected with the cure of leprosy.
385 Pati, 'Order of Legitimacy'.
386 Hunter, *Orissa*, 139.
387 Hunter, *Orissa*, 139. Hunter pointed out that Brahmans had the monopoly in education, which "they kept . . . strictly in their own hands".
388 Hunter, *Orissa*, 104.
389 *Ibid.*, 104.
390 *Ibid.*, 106.
391 *Ibid.*, 108.
392 *Ibid.*, 109.
393 *Ibid.*, 109.
394 *Ibid.*, 109.
395 *Ibid.*, 105.
396 On prisons see: David Arnold, 'The Colonial Prison: Power, Knowledge and Penology in nineteenth-century India', in D. Arnold and D. Hardiman (eds.), *Subaltern Studies VIII*, New Delhi: Oxford University Press, 1994, 148–84; Clare Anderson, 'The Politics of Convict Space: Indian Penal Settlements and the Andaman Islands', in Alison Bashford and C. Strange (eds.), *Isolation: Places and Practices of Exclusion*, London: Routledge, 2003, 40–55. Sanchari Dutta, *Disease and Medicine in Indian Prisons: Confinement in Colonial Bengal, 1860–1910*, PhD Dissertation, University of Oxford, 2008.
397 Hunter, *Orissa*, 110.
398 Nicholas B. Dirks, *The Hollow Crown: Ethnohistory of an Indian Kingdom*, New York: Cambridge University Press, 1987. For a criticism of the "little kingdom" concept, see Hira Singh, 'Colonial and Postcolonial Historiography and the Princely States: Relations of Power and Rituals of Legitimation', in Waltraud Ernst and Biswamoy Pati (eds.), *India's Princely States: People, Princes and Colonialism*, London: Routledge, 2007; New Delhi: Primus, 2009, 15–29.
399 Chandi Prasad Nanda, *Vocalizing Silence: Political Protests in Orissa, 1930–42*, London: Sage, 2008, 172. The numbers provided vary in the sources. The demonstrations soon escalated and a *lathi* charge against 15,000 people took place, followed the next morning by another demonstration of 40,000 people armed with "lathis, bows and arrows, guns, spears, axes, crow-bars etc". B.N. Banerjee, *Dhenkanal Unrest: A Review*, Cuttack: National Publicity Bureau, [n.d. ?1938/9], 4–5, 6. The official line of the British was that "The European force was perfectly inoffensive all through." (p. 8). One of the main concerns for the British related to the involvement of the Kisan movement, a peasant movement supported by the Communist Party of India (CPI).
400 Nanda, *Vocalizing Silence*, 171.

401 National Library Kolkata: Selections From Official Letters and Records Relating to the History of Mayurbhanj, Vol. 2, 1821–1861, Baripada, Mayurbhanj State: Baptist Mission Press, 1943, [Illegible] to Under Secretary to Government of Bengal, 20.3.1861, No 660, paras 1, 3. Incidentally, Indian royalty shared with its European counterparts the prevalence of intrigue: The incumbent Maharaja delayed his installation and receiving of the robe of honour, or Khillut, to avoid the impression that it was given as an award for surrendering his near relation, the Rajah of Porahat. (para. 4).

402 Hunter, *Orissa*, 113.

403 *Ibid.*

404 *Ibid.*

405 Referring to "Mr Stirling's Account" in *Asian Researches* (Vol. xv, pp. 299–305), William Hunter noted: Maratha rule "was fatal to the welfare of the people and the prosperity of the country; and exhibits a picture of misrule, anarchy, weakness, rapacity, and violence combined, which makes one wonder how society can have kept together under so calamitous a tyranny". Hunter, *Orissa*, 32. Andrew Sterling, *An Account (Geographical, Statistical and Historical) of Orissa Proper or Cuttack*, London: John Snow, 1846.

406 D.M. Praharaj, *Tribal Movements and Political History in India: A Case Study From Orissa, 1803–1949*, New Delhi: Inter-India Publications, 1988, 12.

407 Praharaj, *Tribal Movements*, 12–13.

408 Hunter, *Orissa*, 66.

409 Hunter, *Orissa*, 91–2. Quoting Macpherson's Report, Part V, para. 80. Major S.C. Macpherson, *Report Upon the Khonds of the Districts of Ganjam and Cuttack*, Calcutta: 1863[1842].

410 National Library of India, Kolkata: S.C. Bose, *Problem of Orissa*, Calcutta: S.C. Bose, [no date provided], 26–7.

411 Sailendra Nath Sarkar, *Biography of the Maharaja Sri Ram Chandra Bhanj Deo, Feudatory Chief of Mayurbhanj*, Calcutta: Mayurbhanj Estate*, 1918, 24. NB: * "Estate", as in the original source, available in the National Library of India Kolkata.

412 Sarkar, *Biography*, 23. Another British officer, Mr H.P. Wylly, administered the state during Sri Ram Chandra's minority (p. 32), while Mrs Kiddell, by "force of her commanding personality" was central in "forming the character" of the young ruler, giving also "her whole-hearted devotion to the poor lepers of Mayurbhanj". As in the case of Rawenshaw and his protege, the maharaja "later on founded an asylum, of which Mrs. Kiddell was the guiding spirit and manager". P. 41. Service in 'native' states had its career advantages for British staff, while guaranteeing that rulers became enthused with the culture and values of European modernity.

413 Sarkar, *Biography*, 30.

414 *Ibid.*

415 *Ibid.*

416 *Ibid.*

417 *Ibid.*

418 *Ibid.*

419 *Ibid.*

420 There is evidence of patients from British Orissa and Princely states being transferred to institutions in British provinces; their maintenance had to be paid by the states that availed themselves of services outside their jurisdiction.

421 Paul St-Pierre, Leelawati Mohapatra and K.K. Mohapatra, *Ants, Ghosts and Whispering Trees: An Anthology of Oriya Short Stories*, New Delhi: Harper Collins, 2003.

422 Mr Wylly's annual report, Medical Department, 1882/3, quoted in Sarkar, *Biography*, 113.

423 Sarkar, *Biography*, 114.

424 *Ibid.*, 114.

425 *Ibid.*, 115.
426 *Ibid.*, 117.
427 *Ibid.*, 126–7.
428 B. Pati, 'Tatas and the Orissa "Model" of Capitalist "Development"', *Social Scientist*, 34(3), 2006, 37–42.
429 Sri Nilamani Senapati and Nabin Kumar Sahu, *Gazetteer of India: Orissa. Mayurbhanj*, Cuttack: Orissa Government Press, 1967, 82.
430 During the early period of Krishna Chandra Bhanja's reign, from 1867 onwards (Ravenshaw), and from 1882 to 1892 and 1912 to 1920 (Wylly) as heads of the Courts of Ward for Sriram Chandra Bhanja and Purna Chandra Bhanja, respectively.
431 H.K. Mishra, *Famines and Poverty in India*, New Delhi: Ashish, 1991; Biswamoy Pati, *Situating Social History: Orissa, 1800–1997*, New Delhi: Orient Longman, 2001.
432 Senapati and Sahu, *Gazetteer*, 76.
433 *Ibid.*, 75.
434 *Ibid.*, 80.
435 Selva J. Raj, 'Santal Region. India', in Bron Taylor (comp.), *Encyclopedia of Religion and Nature*, Vol. 1, Thoemmes, 2005, 1476–8. Rev. Paul O. Bodding, *Santal Medicine and Connected Folklore*. (Asiatic Society, 1905. British and also Indian authors tend to describe both *ojha* and *dans* as "witches". See for example, Senapati and Sahu, *Gazetteer*, 431. Onkar Prasad, 'Tribal Music: Its Proper Context', in Baidyanath Saraswati (ed.), *Tribal Thought and Culture: Essays in Honour of Surajit Chandra Sinha*, New Delhi: Concept, 1991, 149.
436 Hunter, *Orissa*, 138.
437 *Ibid.*
438 Pati, 'Interrogating Stereotypes', 178.

Index

Adivasis/tribals 7, 9, 45, 55–7, 62, 70,
74–5, 106, 136–7, 140; belief on evil
spirits and leprosy 51; cults of 136;
methods of treating leprosy among 57;
see also smallpox; tribal society
Agrasala 98
agricultural labourers, exploitation of 95
Aiya, Nagam (Dewan) 97, 99–101, 120
All Travancore Sidha Vaydia Sanghom 102
amildar 4, 16, 33–4, 36
Anglo-Indians 106
annual congregations 47, 53; *see also* jatras
anti-colonial mass struggle 68
anti-leprosy campaign (1930) 55–6; *see
also* leprosy
anti-plague measures 19–22; *see also* plague
apothecaries 28, 30, 120
Arnold, David 62; on method of
variolation 65
Arumugum Mudaliar, T.V. 32
Arya Vaidya Samajam, Panikkar on 102
Ashtangahridayam 100–1
assistant surgeons 28–9, 56, 120–1, 124;
abolishing grade of 30
asylum 4, 55–7, 109, 111, 113–16, 120–1,
131; at Adoor 57; and Bengal Leper Act
49; at Cuttack 57; for leper 55–7; for
lunatics 4, 86; of Mysore State 28; in
Oolampura 110; products by inmates of
122; rules and regulations for 115
Ayilyam Thirunal, Maharaja 85
Ayurveda/auyurvedic: dispensaries 100;
drugs production 101; healthcare
providers 120; medicine 99; Pathasala
101; practitioners of 99; system 45,
99–103, 143

Bacteriological Laboratory 40n35
Bamanaghati 55, 71

Bangalore City 13, 15–16, 18–19, 21–2,
31; disinfection arrangements at
Railway Stations 16; plague in 16; strict
measures and public resentments in 22
Baripada 55–6, 139–40
Baripada Leprosy Asylum 56
Bayi, Maharani Lakshmi 86
Bazin, Harve on inoculation 61–2
Bengal Leper Act of 1895 49
Bengal presidency 5
Bennett, James Risdon 49
Benson, P.H. (Brigade-Surgeon Lt.
Colonel) 34–5
Bhanj, Krishna Chandra 55, 139
Bhanja, Maharaja Purna Chandra 140
Bhawanipatana 72
bhoots (ghosts) 70; *see also* evil spirits;
witches (*dans* or *jans*); witchcraft
Bhramaramari Bhandara 52
Bhramaramari plant as medicine 51–2
births and deaths, recording/registration
of 4, 19
Black Town (Indian part of Madras),
lying-in hospital in 94; *see also*
in-patient accommodation
Bose, S.C. 138
Bowring Hospital, Bangalore 4
Bowser, H.C. 139
Breay, Revd C.F. 116–17
British medical approaches and policies 2
British-ruled areas 6–8, 135, 140, 143;
Calicut 101; Madras 9, 117–18
Buckingham, Jane 57
Byabastha Patra 52

camps 13, 18, 20–2; police protection to 19
caste 103–6; inequalities 95; movements
106; reform 9, 90, 94; reform
movements 95

Central Sanitary Board 31–2
Chandramohan, P. 112
chariot festival 47, 136
charitable: dispensaries 73, 137;
    institutions 93, 104
Charity Hospital 89
Charles (Miss) 55
Chemical disinfection 18
Chief Medical Officer 71–2
Chithira Thirunal, Maharaja Sri 106
cholera epidemic 34, 87–8, 120, 135
Christianity, convertion to 95–6, 105
Christian missions 85, 96; *see also* Church
    Missionary Society; missionaries
Christians 55, 88, 92, 105–6, 109
Church Missionary Society 86
City Improvement Committees 33
Civil Disobedience Movement 68
Civil Hospital in Trivandrum 89–90, 98,
    110
civilizing mission 7, 9, 45, 47, 56, 62, 67,
    70, 75, 134, 136
colonial: medical establishment 47, 53,
    55–6; medicine 1–2; psychiatry 2,
    83–4; vaccination policy 62, 68, 74;
    Vaccination Programme 72, 75
colonialism 5, 7, 62, 64, 66, 74, 84
communal strife 106
communicable diseases 14, 32
compounders 54, 56, 120, 124, 140
Compulsory vaccination Act 34–5
confinement 45, 49, 51, 54, 57, 113–14,
    131, 139; *see also* lepers
Congress Ministry 50; installation of 68
contagious diseases 87; prevention of
    26; *see also* disinfection; sanitation;
    vaccination
Countess of Reading's Women's Fund 140
County Asylums Act of 1845 131
Cox, Jeffrey 94
Cromwell 87
Cuttack Leprosy Asylum 50
Cuttack Medical College 53

Dalhousie (Lord) 86
Dalits 57
darbars 6–9, 50, 53–5, 57, 70–1, 73–4, 142;
    physicians of 87, 104, 113–16, 120, 122–3
Dasara Session 13
deaths 4–5, 13–16, 18–19, 21–2, 32, 34–6,
    52, 71, 74, 117, 129; of Father Damien
    46, 48–9; on influenza 36; by plague 20;
    and secret burial 20; from smallpox 35
Deo, Krishna Chandra Bhanj 55

Deo, Purna Chandra Bhanja 141
depressed castes 105–6; *see also* Dalits;
    pana (untouchables)
Deputy Inspector of Vaccination 33, 36
Deputy Sanitary Commissioner 32
Desai: on Christian mission 96; on land
    reform 86; on Travancore 96
devasoms (Devaswom, religious
    institutions) 96–9
devil dancing, as treatment for insanity
    112, 121
dharmabhumi 95
Dharma Pinnu (goddess of smallpox) 63,
    75, 76n16
Dhenkanal 2, 5, 73, 136–7, 139, 141; as
    most civilized 137; Nanda on 137
Digby, A. 119
discrimination: against caste 106; against
    leprosy 45; *see also pana* (untouchables)
Diseases of the Bible, The 49
disinfection: of houses 15, 22, 24n25; of
    infected persons 18
dispensaries 4, 8, 28–30, 33, 53, 72, 90–1,
    99, 103–4, 120, 139–40; at Bangripsi
    56; Banpur 54; in Mysore State 28;
    at Satpara 54; Udala 56; *see also*
    charitable, dispensaries
District Plague Officers 16
District Sanitary Board 32
drinking water sources, chlorination of 4
Duff, Grant 85
Dufferin, Lady 29
Dufferin philanthropic movement 29
Durbar Surgeon 27

East India Company 6, 86
education, higher branch of 8, 91
electrotherapy 127–8
English East India Company 6
enslavement, abolition of 8
epidemic 4–5, 13–16, 20–2, 26, 33–7,
    64, 72, 74; absence of 73; evacuating
    andlocalities of 22
Epidemic Disease Hospital 5; in Bangalore
    14, 32
Epidemic Diseases Regulation (1897) 4, 32
Esmonde White, H.P. (Surgeon Major)
    114–15
European: Medical Officers 27; and
    methods of sexual segregation 57; and
    racial prejudice 106
Evangelical Society 55
evil spirits 45, 51, 88; *see also bhoots*
    (ghosts); witches (dans or jans)

exploitation 2, 8, 66, 95, 133–4, 138, 141–2; *see also* agricultural labourers, exploitation of
exterior castes 105–6
Ezhavas/Iluvas (low caste/untouchables) *vydians* 95, 99, 112

fairs and festivals 15; sanitation and 118
family planning 5
famines 48, 53, 96, 133, 135–6, 141; relief works in Bengal 94; *see also* Naanka Durbikhya-famine of 1866
Fawcett, Henry (Sir) 87
female infanticide 107
female school, in Calcutta 94
fevers 61, 87
Finsen, Niels 128
Fort Hospital, Namboodiri patients and 90
fraudulent practices 124; *see also* quacks

Gandhi, Mahatma 106
Ganjam or Shahar Ganjam 21, 66; riots in 21–2
Gantayita 52
gender discrimination 107–9
gendered treatment pattern 128
Gillespie, R.D. 125
Government Ayurveda College 101
Government of India Act of 1919 68
government services 93, 116, 125
Grant, Charles 94
Grant Duff, M.E. (Sir) 85
grant-in-aid 103
Griffith, M. 84–5
Gupta, Purna Chandra 140
Guru, Narayana 99
Gustafson, Donald Rudolf 20

Habermas, Juergen 96
Hacker, T.H. 94
Haliya Brahmins 74
Hansen, discovery of leprosy bacillus (*Mycobacterium leprae*) 46–7
Hardiman, D. 63
Harrison, Mark, on smallpox vaccination 66
Hayagrivacharya 20
health services 4–5, 68, 134, 137, 142
Henderson, D.K. 125
Hinduization 51–2, 62, 74
Hindus 7, 49, 62–3, 75, 94, 105–6, 108–9, 139; of high caste 7, 105, 109; purification of 106
hospital assistants 16, 27–9, 120, 139–40

hospitalization 21–2; opposition to 20
hospitals 3–5, 8, 20–2, 28, 71, 90–1, 103–4, 112, 120–1, 123, 131–2; categorization among admission staff in 105; funding for 26; for infectious diseases 32; in Mysore State 28; seen as jails 20
Howell, J.Z. 65
Hunter, W.W. 134–8, 142
Huzzoor Cutcherry [Secretariat] Hospital 90

immunization services 4; *see also* vaccination
Indian: royalty 3; rulers 1–3, 9
Indian Army Medical Corps (IAMC) 124
Indian Mental Hospital at Ranchi 108
Indian middle classes 7
Indian Plague Commission Report 22
Indian Rebellion, Mutiny of 1857 85–6
indigenous: hospital in Mysore 39n28; medicine and Vaidyasalas 99–103; practices 26–7
influenza pandemic 36–7
inoculation 18–20, 61–2, 65–6, 68, 74–5; and Brahmin 65; and leprosy Gustafson on 20; non-tribal as 64–5
in-patient accommodation 103–4
Ismail, Mirza M. 33
isolation/forcible confinement, European experience of 21, 46–7, 54
Iyappan, Madaven 114–16

jatras 20, 33, 136; *see also* annual congregations; Puri Jagannatha (ratha jatras Puri Jagannatha)
Jeffrey, R. 86
Johnson, A.S. 88, 121–5, 132
Jopp, W. (Chief Engineer) 116–17

Kakar, Sanjeev 57
Kalahandi 2, 5, 72, 133
Kandhas 63–7, 75
Keonjhar 2, 5, 50–2, 54, 57, 71–2; Anandapur clinic in 54; darbars engagement of 53, 57; leaf manuscripts on leprosy treatment in 51; population of 54
Khalid, A. 88
King, Surgeon Major 35
King Institute of Guindy 68
Kols 135
Kooiman 94–5
K.R. Hospital 4–5

Kumara Pillai, V. 125
Kuttia Kandhas 63

laboratory 32
La Bouchardiere, M. 117
Lady Curzon Hospital, Bangalore 4
land: commodification of 95; ownership
of 95
land acquisition legislation 33, 40n41
land revenue 86; of Balasore 5; of Nilgiri
state 6; settlements of 6
lano-line paste 35; *see also* vaccination
Leper Clinic, Mayurbhanj 55
lepers 2, 48–50, 53–5, 57, 120; asylums
for 4; compulsory confinement of 45–6;
as criminalization of 47; at pilgrimage
sites 47; poor as 48, 50; prohibition on
49; prosecution of 46; strike in Cochin
57; Waters on 53; WHO estimation of
60n58
Leper's Act of 1898 49
leprosy: adivasi healing systems for
50–5; Bhramaramari plant as a cure for
51, 59n32; Brahminical Hinduism on
45; Chaulmogra oil for 45–7, 54; and
colonial authorities 47; criminalization
of 49; detection of 56; Foucault
on 45; germ theory for 46, 55; and
hereditary theory 46; and insatiable
sexual desire 46; Islam on 45; Jesus
'curing' 45; Jews as carriers of 46;
and Muslims 48; 'Otherization' of
45; and stereotypes 45–6; stigma and
discrimination against 45; treatment
for 51; vaccine for 45
Leprosy Asylums 4, 50, 54–6, 120; at
Baripada 56; *see also* asylum; Leper
Clinic, Mayurbhanj
Leung, Angela K.C. 61; method of
variolation 61
Lewis, Aubrey 125
local: funds 28–9; medical service 27–8;
people, training of 73
London Missionary Society 88
lower caste women, and breasts covering 95
Low/Haliya Brahmins 74
Lukose, Mary Poonen Dr. 107
Lunacy Regulation of 1904/5 112
lunatic asylum 2, 4, 30, 91, 111–12,
114–15, 117, 119–21, 128, 130, 137;
as hospital for mental diseases 121;
and hospital in Bangalore 39n15;
medicalization of admission and
discharge 115; at Trivandrum 109–17

lunatic patients 28, 109, 113–14, 116;
statistics, trends and 128–33; treatment
of patients, classification and 125–8
lymph production centres 69

MacKenzie, G.T. 120
Macpherson, S.C. (Major) 138
Madava (Rao) Raw, (Dewan) 15, 20–2, 84,
87, 98
Madhava Rao, T. 86
Madhava Rao, V.P. 15, 21
Madras government 8, 27, 122
Madras Medical College 122
Madras Medical Subordinates, in Mysore 27
Mahomedan vydians 101
Mapother, Edward 83, 132–3
Marthas Hospital, Bangalore 5
Mastan Brahmins 68
Mateer, Samuel (Rev.) 92, 94–5, 98; on
Muhammedans 88
maternity hospitals 5, 90, 120
matrons 120, 124; *see also* midwives
Maudsley Mental Hospital 83, 121, 125,
132–3
Mayurbhanj 2, 5, 50, 55–7, 70–1, 138–41;
health system in 56, 138; population of
134; society of 138; starvation in 141
medical: education 102; establishments
27, 67, 70–1, 74, 104; practitioner 103,
120; provision 103–6; services 2, 26–7,
83, 100–1, 107–8, 119; subordinates 27,
87, 118
medical department 8, 27, 30, 73, 87,
91–4, 96, 98, 102, 123–5, 139–40;
reorganization of 8
medical institutions 2, 4, 27–8, 30,
71–2, 100, 120, 124–5, 129–30, 133;
popularity of 71; in Travancore 131
Medical Officers 14–15, 27, 30, 53, 71, 87,
91, 103, 115–16, 119, 124; categories of
27; complaints against 123; as local 27
Medical Practitioners' Bill 102
medical reforms 92; and funding priorities
92–4; by "Travancore's Cromwell" 87
medical schools 5, 29, 140; *see also*
medical institutions
medicine as 'tool of empire' 1
Menon, P.K.K. 89–90, 101
mental health 8–9, 84, 135–6, 139–42;
Mapother on 132; in Orissan states 9;
Western-style 119
mental hospitals 125, 130–1; admissions
to 109, 131; by British 83; in Ceylon 83;
with 'chronic cases' 133; classification

scheme at 125; and employment of nurses 125; in Indian Princely states 83; of the Indian Princely states 83; Johnson on 123–4; at Mysore 9; nurses employed in 125; over representation of caste Hindus in 109; in Princely Mysore 9, 131, 133; Ranchi, caste Hindus over-represented in 109; in Travancore 108–9; in Trivandrum 127

Mental Treatment Act 123

Messrs Jacob Taliat 125

Meyer, Swiss-American Adolf 125

midwives 28–9, 101, 120, 124

Minto Eye Hospital 5

Mishra, M.M. 88, 133

missionaries 8, 46, 49–50, 55, 92, 94–5, 112; and caste reform 94–6; initiatives of 94; and leprosy 50, 55; and Munro 86; and reforms 94; against slavery and caste discrimination 86; and Travancore public health 9

Mission of Lepers, The 55

Mission of Lepers in India 50

modernity 7, 98, 134, 139, 142–3; Pati on 142

modern psychiatry 130

modern Travancore 98

Montagu, Mary Wortley 61

Municipalities of Bangalore and Mysore 22, 35

Munro, John 86, 94

Murajapam festival 90

Muslims/Muhammedans 3, 48, 89, 106, 109; and anti-plague measures 20; and leprosy 48–9

Mysore Cities 15, 19, 31; birth control clinics in 5; disinfection at Railway Stations 16; strict measures and public resentments in 22

Mysore Epidemic Diseases Regulation Act in 1897 14

Mysore Medical School, Bangalore 29

Mysore Public Service 28

Mysore Representative Assembly 4, 13, 26, 28, 33

Mysore State 3–5, 16, 21–2, 24n14, 25n40, 29; dispensaries in 28; as 'model state' 4; population of 13; public health administration in 27–31; sanitation 27–33

Mysore Village Sanitary Regulation (1898) 33

Naanka Durbikhya-famine of 1866 53, 141

Nagalkata (a village) Mission 55

Nair, Velayudhan 122

Nairs/Nayars 86, 89, 92, 95, 98; revolt by 86

Nambudiri doctors 100

Nanda, Chandi Prasad 137

Nanoo Pillay, N. (Dewan) 114

Napier, Lord Francis 85, 99

Narayanen, Madhav 114–15

native medicines 99–100, 103

native vydians 99

natural resources, appeal to exploitation of 3, 8, 91, 134, 142

Nayar Brigade, hospital for 91

Needham, J., practice of variolation of 61

Nellikaray Vedic College 114

Neyyoor mission hospital 94

Nilacanta Pillai, N.P. 121

Nilgiri 2, 5, 73

Non-Cooperation Movement 68

Norman White, F. 36

occupational industries 128

Oolampara [Ulampara], institution at 121; *see also* mental hospitals

Ootuparas 96, 98–9; allocation of 98

oppression 134–5, 137–8, 141 on Hindu communities 105

Orissa Engineering College in Bihar 140

Orissan states 2–3, 5–9, 133–42; annexation of 5; colonization of 62; Pati on 133

Orissa States Peoples Conference 134

Oriya middle class 56

outcastes 7–8, 74, 89–90, 94, 105–6, 136, 140

out-patients 89–91, 103, 105–7, 129; medical treatment at grant-in-aid institutions 104; Western government-sponsored institutions 104

Padmanabhaswamy Pagoda 98

Paikas 64, 66

Palace Hospital 90

palm-leaf manuscripts 51–2

pana (untouchables) 63, 68, 73–4; as vaccinators 73

Panikkar, K.N. 99, 102

Pati, B. 133, 135–6, 142

Pati, Maheshwar 56

peasant movements 137

Pennoo, Joogah 63

permanent settlement 6, 9, 97

Phipps Psychiatric Clinic at Baltimore 125

Pillai, Kumary 125

Pillai, Venu 121

Pillai, V.K. 125, 127

Pillay, V.V. 110, 112–13, 121
plague 2, 5, 13–16, 18–22, 34, 37, 88,
    135; administrative measures against
    14–19; in Bangalore 13; in Bombay 13;
    death in Bombay City by 23n11; deaths
    by 16, 22; hospital for 14, 22; at Hubli
    13; measures 22; and public resistance
    19–21; Seshadri Iyer on 13
Plague Commissioner 15, 21–2, 32
Plague Department 15
Planter's Hospital at Ashambi 91
political movements 9, 106, 134, 142
Poonen, E. 107–8
Poonen, Mary 107–8
poverty 133
poverty schools 8, 91
practitioners 2, 99, 101–2, 139
Praharaj, D.M. 138
prajamandal peasant movements 73, 134, 137
precautionary measures 14–15, 22
preventive measures 14–15, 19; *see also*
    disinfection; sanitation; segregation
Princely darbars 7
Princely Kochin 85
Princely states/native states 1–3, 5–6,
    38nn5–6, 50–1, 53–4, 57, 61–2,
    66, 68–9, 74, 83–4, 96; *Dhenkanal*
    73–4; *Gangpur* 70; *Kalahandi* 72–3;
    Keonjhar 71–2; of Keonjhar 50, 53–4;
    Mayurbhanj 70–1; Mysore 4, 22, 133;
    Nilgiri 73; of Orissa 2, 50–1, 57, 61–2
Promin, discovery of 57
Province of Orissa 62, 67, 135; formation
    of 54, 68
Prussian Lutheran William Ringeltaube 94
psychiatrists 125; *see also* Trivandrum
public health 2, 4–8, 26–7, 31, 33, 35, 49,
    109; measures on 26, 117, 140; statistics
    118
Public Health Institute 5, 32
public resentment 20–1, 88
Pulney Andy Dr. 118
Puri, as centre of leprosy 47
Puri Jagannatha (ratha jatras Puri
    Jagannatha) 136
Puri Leprosy House 49

quacks 100
Quilon and Shencotta roads, construction
    of 93
Quit India Movement 68

race 106
Raghunandan 107

railway medical inspection stations 14
Rajkumar College, Raipur 140
Rama Raw, T. (Dewan) 115
Ramayyan Dalwa (Rama Iyen) 98
Ramusack 84, 86
Ranchi Indian Mental Hospital 109
Rao, Achut 20
Ravenshaw, T.E. 139; on Srinath Bhanja
    141
Ravenshaw College 140
relief measures 5, 20, 36
religious welfare institutions and Brahmin
    privileges 96–9
re-vaccinations 34, 67–9, 72–4
revenue collection 95, 135
Revenue Commissioner 32
revitalization movement 102
Roberts, Frederick (Lord) 7–8, 85
Rockefeller Foundation 8
Roman Catholic Mission 55
Ross, Aeneas Mcleod Dr. 87–92
Roy, Juggoo Mohun on leprosy and
    Muslims 48
royalty 49; degrading treatment of lower
    and outcastes under 7; Hindu 3; Indian
    3; of Travancore 104
rural sanitary measures 118

sacrifices 63, 70, 88; *see also* evil spirits;
    witchcraft
Sadr Hospital, Orissa State 72
salary, of Medical officers 27–30
Sanatoria 91
sanitary administration 27, 31–3, 37
Sanitary Commissioner 15, 31–4, 36, 117,
    119
Sanitary Engineer 31–2
sanitation 4, 13, 19, 26–7, 31–3, 103–4,
    117; Annual Sanitary Report 32; control
    measures 88; reforms on 5, 26, 31, 88
Santals/Santhals 51, 64, 135; *see also*
    smallpox
Sarkar, S.N. 140
Sastri, Sashia (Dewan) 97
Schizophrenic Reaction Type 123
scholarships to students 29
School of Tropical Medicine, Calcutta 55
segregation 5, 14–15, 18, 21–2, 46, 49–52,
    57, 137; of lepors 45–6; opposition to
    20; social 106
semi-nomadic peoples 9
Senior Surgeons 15, 29–31, 34–6
Seshadri Iyer, K. 13–14, 28, 31
Seshayya Sastri, A. 97

Shanars 95
Sharma, S.P. 133–4
sick nurses 120
Siddha 102–3, 143
Simpson, James Dr. 108, 123
Sirkar Pattom 97
Sitala (goddess of smallpox) 63–5, 74–5; inoculationa and 68; pana (ritualistic drink to) 63; *see also* Dharma Pinnu (goddess of smallpox)
smallpox 5, 34–5, 50, 61–7, 70–4, 135; Arnold on 65; broke out in Kurumkel 70; and colonial establishment 65–9; death by 61, 71; eradication of 75; lost label of epidemic 72; medicines for 64; and tribals 62–4; vaccination against 8, 38n6, 61–2, 65–6, 68, 71, 75, 78n52
Southern-Mahratta Railway 14
Sri Narayana Dharma Paripalan (SNDP) 112
Sri Ramakrishna Ashram, dispensary, Vakkom 103
State Leper Asylum, Baripada 55
Stewart, W.D., on leprosy and famine of 1866 48
Sudras 98, 100–1
Sultan, Tipu 86
surgeons 27–9, 65, 124–5
suzerainty 1
Syrian Christians 95; as *vydians* 101

Talcher darbar 6
Tata Iron and Steel Company, Sakchi 140
Temple Entry Proclamation (1931) 106
temple services, and low castes oppression 92
Thomson, H. (Major) 120
Towns Improvement and Conservancy Regulation 117
Travancore 3, 7–9, 84–7; as Dhurma Raj 98; joining Indian Union 7; as "land of charity" 98; medical reforms and social stratification 87–92; middle class of 9; social welfare measures of 85; untouchables in 95
Travancore Mental Hospital 133
Travancore State Manual 113, 121
treatment 14, 18, 20, 46–7, 51–4, 90–1, 100–2, 110, 113–14, 121–2, 127–8; of leprosy 51, 54, 57; method of and fear of injection 57; by ojhas 142; in Western-style institutions 142
tribal society 63–4, 70, 75; and loyalty 136; oral tradition of 52, 62; and small pox 62; *see also* Adivasis/tribals
tribute or *peshkush* 6

Trivandrum (Thiruvananthapuram) 85; psychiatric provision at 119–25
Trivandrum Mental Hospital 130; *see also* Oolampara [Ulampara], institution at
Trollope 104
Tropical School of Medicine, Calcutta 54

Unani Vaidyasala, Menon on 101
unprotected children 33, 36; survey on 35
untouchables 68, 74, 95, 105; temples and roads usage and 95; *see also* Dalits; *pana* (untouchables)
upper-caste mutiny 86; *see also* Indian Rebellion, Mutiny of 1857; Nairs/ Nayars, revolt by
Utkal Sahitya Parishad (Orissa Literary Association) 140

vaccination 4, 8, 25n31, 26, 33–6, 64–75, 86, 94, 104, 117–18, 135; campaigns for 88; expenditure of 71; fees of 68; as free and compulsory 72; in Mysore state 33–6; policy for 74; for smallpox 67; supervision of 32
vaccination programme 33, 69, 71, 74
Vaccination Regulation Act of 1906 4
vaccinators 33–6, 65–8, 70–1, 73–5, 118; attack on 68; female/women as 70, 73–4; Pana (untouchables) as 73
Vaccine Depot at Namkum 73–4
Vaccine Institute 5, 35, 68–9
vaidyans 100
vaidyasalas 99–101, 103, 120
Variar, P.S. 101–2
Varma, King Marthanda 96
Varma, Maharaja Marthanda 98
Varma, Rama 85
Velu Pillai, T.K. 113
vexatious taxes 84
Victoria Hospital 5, 29, 39n22
Victoria Memorial Institute, Baripada 140
Vijayindra Rao, R. 27
village functionaries (Patels) 35–6
Village Improvement Committees 33
Village Sanitary Act 8
Village Sanitation Regulation (1898) 14
Visakham Thirunal, Maharaja 85
Visvesvaraya, M. (Dewan) 36

Ward Officers 16
Waters, E.E. 53; putrid fish theory of 54
Western: healthcare 104; medical department 103; medical facilities in Travancore 120; medical systems 49

Western medicine 1–2, 13, 20, 26, 98, 102, 139; and affiliated institutions 104
Western Star, The 92
Western-style institutions 139
White, Esmonde 115
witchcraft 51, 70
witches (*dans* or *jans*) 64, 70, 75, 142

Wodeyars 27, 37
Women and Children's Hospital, Trivandrum 107, 123
work therapy 110
Wylly, H.P. 139–41

zymotic or preventable diseases 87

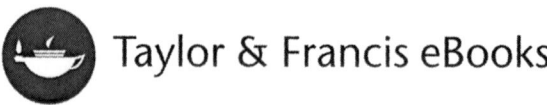

Taylor & Francis eBooks

Helping you to choose the right eBooks for your Library

Add Routledge titles to your library's digital collection today. Taylor and Francis ebooks contains over 50,000 titles in the Humanities, Social Sciences, Behavioural Sciences, Built Environment and Law.

Choose from a range of subject packages or create your own!

Benefits for you

» Free MARC records
» COUNTER-compliant usage statistics
» Flexible purchase and pricing options
» All titles DRM-free.

Benefits for your user

» Off-site, anytime access via Athens or referring URL
» Print or copy pages or chapters
» Full content search
» Bookmark, highlight and annotate text
» Access to thousands of pages of quality research at the click of a button.

REQUEST YOUR **FREE** INSTITUTIONAL TRIAL TODAY

Free Trials Available
We offer free trials to qualifying academic, corporate and government customers.

eCollections – Choose from over 30 subject eCollections, including:

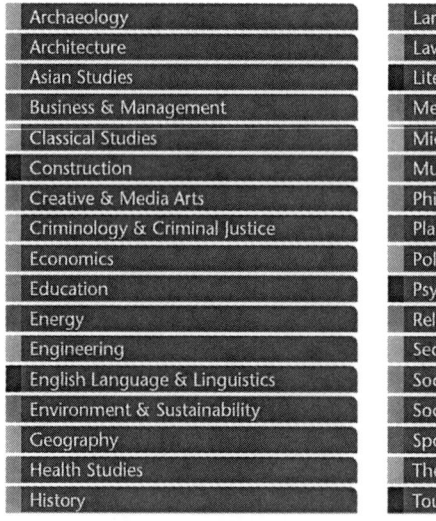

Archaeology	Language Learning
Architecture	Law
Asian Studies	Literature
Business & Management	Media & Communication
Classical Studies	Middle East Studies
Construction	Music
Creative & Media Arts	Philosophy
Criminology & Criminal Justice	Planning
Economics	Politics
Education	Psychology & Mental Health
Energy	Religion
Engineering	Security
English Language & Linguistics	Social Work
Environment & Sustainability	Sociology
Geography	Sport
Health Studies	Theatre & Performance
History	Tourism, Hospitality & Events

For more information, pricing enquiries or to order a free trial, please contact your local sales team:
www.tandfebooks.com/page/sales

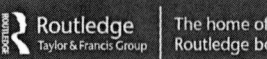